Q000673

HPNA PALLIATIVE NURSING MANUALS

Series edited by Betty R. Ferrell, RN, PhD, MA, FAAN, FPCN, CHPN

Volume 1: Structure and Processes of Care

Volume 2: Physical Aspects of Care: Pain and Gastrointestinal Symptoms

Volume 3: Physical Aspects of Care: Nutritional, Dermatologic, Neurologic and Other Symptoms

Volume 4: Pediatric Palliative Care

Volume 5: Social Aspects of Care

Volume 6: Spiritual, Religious, and Existential Aspects of Care and Cultural Aspects

Volume 7: Care of the Patient at the End of Life

Volume 8: Ethical and Legal Aspects

HPNA PALLIATIVE NURSING MANUALS

Structure and Processes of Care

Edited by

Betty R. Ferrell, RN, PhD, MA, FAAN, FPCN, CHPN

Professor and Director
Department of Nursing Research and Education
City of Hope Comprehensive Cancer Center
Duarte, California

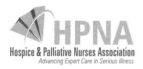

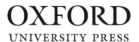

OXFORD
UNIVERSITY PRESS

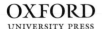

OXFORD
UNIVERSITY PRESS

Oxford University Press is a department of the University of
Oxford. It furthers the University's objective of excellence in research,
scholarship, and education by publishing worldwide.

Oxford   New York
Auckland   Cape Town   Dar es Salaam   Hong Kong   Karachi
Kuala Lumpur   Madrid   Melbourne   Mexico City   Nairobi
New Delhi   Shanghai   Taipei   Toronto

With offices in
Argentina   Austria   Brazil   Chile   Czech Republic   France   Greece
Guatemala   Hungary   Italy   Japan   Poland   Portugal   Singapore
South Korea   Switzerland   Thailand   Turkey   Ukraine   Vietnam

Oxford is a registered trademark of Oxford University Press
in the UK and certain other countries.

Published in the United States of America by
Oxford University Press
198 Madison Avenue, New York, NY 10016

Library of Congress Cataloging-in-Publication Data
Structure and processes of care / edited by Betty R. Ferrell.
p. ; cm. —(HPNA palliative nursing manuals ; volume 1)
"Content for this series was derived primarily from the Oxford Textbook of Palliative
Nursing (4th edition, 2015), edited by Betty R. Ferrell, Nessa Coyle, Judith A. Paice.
The Textbook contains more extensive content and references so users of this Palliative
Nursing Manual are encouraged to use the Textbook as an additional resource."—Preface.
Includes bibliographical references and index.
ISBN 978–0–19–022375–5 (alk. paper)
I. Ferrell, Betty, editor.   II. Oxford textbook of palliative nursing. 4th edition. 2014.
Based on (expression): III. Series: HPNA palliative nursing manuals ; v. 1.
[DNLM: 1. Hospice and Palliative Care Nursing.   2. Palliative Care.   3. Terminal Care.
WY 152.3]
R726.8
616.02'9—dc23
2014036629

9 8 7 6 5 4 3 2 1
Printed in the United States of America
on acid-free paper

Contents

Preface

This is the first volume of a new series being published by Oxford University Press in collaboration with the Hospice and Palliative Nurses Association. The intent of this series is to provide palliative care nurses with quick reference guides to each of the key domains of palliative care. The volumes mirror the domains established by the National Consensus Project for Quality Palliative Care (NCP), as well as one volume devoted specifically to pediatric palliative care. The series will include:

Volume 1: Structure and Processes of Care—overview of palliative nursing care, review of NCP guidelines and practical tools to use in starting and maintaining palliative care programs

Volume 2: Physical Aspects of Care: Pain and Gastrointestinal Symptoms—pain and other physical symptoms, assessment tools, pharmacology, and patient teaching

Volume 3: Physical Aspects of Care: Nutritional, Dermatologic, Neurologic and Other Symptoms—nutrition and genitourinary symptom management, assessment tools, pharmacology, and patient teaching

Volume 4: Pediatric Palliative Care—key areas of pediatric palliative care, such as pain and symptom management, communication with children based on development level, and key assessment tools

Volume 5: Social Aspects of Care—support of family caregivers and bereavement support

Volume 6: Spiritual, Religious, and Existential Aspects of Care and Cultural Aspects—spiritual care and cultural assessment tools

Volume 7: Care of the Patient at the End of Life—including physical symptoms, discontinuing life support, family caregiver support, and practical tools such as comfort orders and protocols

Volume 8: Ethical and Legal Aspects—to include decision tools, case studies, and models of analysis of ethical dilemmas

Content for this series was derived primarily from the *Oxford Textbook of Palliative Nursing* (4th edition, 2015), which is also edited by Betty Ferrell, Nessa Coyle, and Judith Paice, the editors of this series. The Contributors identified in each volume are the authors of chapters in the *Oxford Textbook of Palliative Nursing* from which the content was selected for this volume. The Textbook contains more extensive content and references, so users of these Palliative Nursing Manuals are encouraged to use the Textbook as an additional resource.

This first volume lays out the structures and processes that are necessary to support quality palliative care. Future volumes will focus on individual aspects of this care.

We are grateful to all palliative care nurses who are contributing to the advancement of care for seriously ill patients and families. Remarkable progress has occurred over the past 30 years in this field, and nurses have been central to that progress. Our hope is that this series offers an additional tool to build the care delivery system we strive for.

Contributors

Romina Arceo, ANP-C

Nurse Practitioner of Pain and
  Palliative Care
Department of Pain Medicine and
  Palliative Care
Beth Israel Medical Center
New York, New York

Marie Bakitas, PhD

Marie L. O'Koren Endowed Chair
  and Professor of Nursing
UAB School of Nursing
The University of Alabama at
  Birmingham
Birmingham, Alabama

Marilyn Bookbinder, RN, PhD

Department of Pain Medicine and
  Palliative Care
Beth Israel Medical Center
New York, New York

**Joan G. Carpenter, MN,
CRNP, NP-C, GNP-BC,
ACHPN, PhD**

Patricia G. Archbold Predoctoral
  Scholar and Doctor of
  Philosophy Student
College of Nursing
University of Utah
Salt Lake City, Utah
Nurse Practitioner
Coastal Hospice and Palliative Care
Berlin, Maryland

**Patrick J. Coyne, MSN, APRN,
FAAN, FPCN**

Clinical Director of the Thomas
  Palliative Care Unit
Virginia Commonwealth University
Massey Cancer Center
Richmond, Virginia

**Constance Dahlin, ANP-BC,
ACHPN, FPCN, FAAN**

Clinical Director
Palliative Care Service
Massachusetts General Hospital
Boston, Massachusetts

**Mary Ersek, PhD, RN,
FPCN, FAAN**

Director of National PROMISE
  Center
Philadelphia Veterans Affairs
  Medical Center
Associate Professor
University of Pennsylvania School
  of Nursing
Philadelphia, Pennsylvania

Laurie J. Lyckholm, MD

Department of Hematology/
  Oncology
Virginia Commonwealth University
Massey Cancer Center
Richmond, Virginia

**Patricia Maani-Fogelman,
DNP**

Department of Palliative Medicine
Geisinger Medical Center
Danville, Pennsylvania

Jennifer McAdam, RN, PhD

Assistant Professor of Nursing
Samuel Merritt University
Oakland, California

Kathleen Puntillo, RN, PhD, FAAN, FCCM
Professor of Nursing
Department of Physiological
    Nursing
University of California,
    San Francisco
San Francisco, California

Thomas J. Smith, MD, FACP, FASCO
Professor of Palliative Medicine and
    Oncology
Johns Hopkins Medicine
Baltimore, Maryland

Pamela Stitzlein Davies, MS, ARNP, ACHPN
Nurse Practitioner
Palliative & Supportive Care
    Service
Seattle Cancer Care Alliance
Seattle, Washington

Chapter 1

National Consensus Project for Quality Palliative Care

Constance Dahlin

The mission of the National Consensus Project for Quality Palliative Care (NCP) is to create clinical practice guidelines to improve and ensure the quality of palliative care in the United States. The NCP's *Clinical Practice Guidelines for Quality Palliative Care,* published in 2004,[1] had a three-pronged goal: (1) to promote quality and reduce variation in new and existing programs, (2) to develop and encourage continuity of care across settings, and (3) to facilitate collaborative partnerships among palliative care programs, community hospices, and a wide range of other healthcare delivery settings. The eight domains of the guidelines are presented in this chapter and listed in Box 1.1.

The *Clinical Practice Guidelines* offer a framework for the future of palliative care. Their purpose is to serve as a manual or blueprint to create new programs, guide developing programs, and set high expectations for excellence in existing programs. The guidelines set ideal practices and goals that palliative care services should strive to attain, rather than minimally acceptable practices. Because the guidelines were not associated with a regulatory body or reimbursement process, they were voluntary. They aimed to achieve the following:

- Facilitate the development and continuing improvement of clinical palliative care programs providing care to patients and families with life-threatening or debilitating illness
- Establish uniformly accepted definitions of the essential elements in palliative care that promote quality, consistency, and reliability of these services

---

Box 1.1 Eight Domains of Care Developed by the National Consensus Project

Domain 1: Structure and Processes of Care
Domain 2: Physical Aspects of Care
Domain 3: Psychological and Psychiatric Aspects of Care
Domain 4: Social Aspects of Care
Domain 5: Spiritual, Religious, and Existential Aspects of Care
Domain 6: Cultural Aspects of Care
Domain 7: Care of the Patient at the End of Life
Domain 8: Ethical and Legal Aspects of Care

- Establish national goals for access to quality palliative care
- Foster performance measurement and quality improvement initiatives in palliative care services
- Foster continuity of palliative care across settings (i.e., home, residential care, rehabilitation, hospital, and hospice)[1]

Basic assumptions about palliative care were constructed. First, palliative care services would adhere to established standards and requirements for healthcare quality, such as safety, effective leadership, medical record keeping, and error reduction. Second, palliative care programs would observe established professional and organizational codes of ethics. Third, the guidelines would continue to evolve and be revised to integrate changes in professional practice, the evidence base, and healthcare reform. Fourth, the consensus process would continue ensuring representation of a broad range of professionals and disciplines. This process would guarantee that the guidelines would continue to promote the highest quality of clinical palliative care services across the healthcare continuum. Fifth, the guidelines would distinguish between specialty palliative care and primary palliative care. Primary palliative care could be incorporated in any discipline and included basic pain and symptom management and communication skills. Specific palliative care qualifications would continue to be delineated by specialty organizations granting professional credentials and programmatic accreditation. Sixth, there was a core assumption that ongoing professional palliative care education would occur and include the knowledge, attitudes, and skills required to deliver quality palliative care across the domains established in the document.[1]

The response to the document was very positive from the professional community, and the NCP guidelines were subsequently endorsed by many organizations and broadly disseminated.

In 2005, the structure of the NCP moved to a collaborative governance structure under the Coalition of Hospice and Palliative Care. In 2006, the National Quality Forum (NQF) used the *Clinical Practice Guidelines* to form the basis of their document, *A National Framework for Palliative and Hospice Care Quality Measurement and Reporting.*[2] The mission of the NQF is to "improve American healthcare through the endorsement of the consensus-based national standards for measurement and public reporting of healthcare performance data. The goal is to maintain meaningful information about the care delivery such as safety, benefit, patient centeredness, equality, and efficiency of healthcare." The NQF adoption of the NCP guidelines was significant because the goal of its document was to formulate palliative care standards and preferred practices with implications for reimbursement, internal and external quality measurement, regulation, and accreditation.[2] See Box 1.2 for a listing of the NCP clinical practice guidelines and the corresponding NQF preferred practices.

In 2009, five years after the initial release of the *Clinical Practice Guidelines,* the landscape of palliative care had changed. The number of palliative care and hospice programs had grown substantially. Palliative care was being discussed in healthcare reform. It was necessary that the

Box 1.2 Nursing Applications of the Clinical Practice Guidelines

Domain 1: Structure and Processes of Care

1. All nurses should receive education in primary palliative care in undergraduate, graduate programs, and doctoral programs.
2. All nurses should pursue continuing education in primary palliative care.
3. All nurses should receive an orientation in primary palliative care that includes attitudes, knowledge, and skills in the domains of palliative care. This includes basic pain and symptom assessment and management, basic communication skills around advanced illness, ethical principles, grief and bereavement, family and community resources, and hospice care (philosophy, eligibility).
4. All nurses, particularly specialty hospice and palliative nurses, should work with an interdisciplinary team, which may include a variety of disciplines.
5. Specialty hospice and palliative nurses should have regularly scheduled and organized support for their palliative care work and designated meetings to discuss their work.
6. Specialty hospice and palliative nurses should be certified in hospice and palliative care. Certification is available for the Nursing Assistant, Licensed Practical/Vocational Nurse, Registered Nurse, and Advanced Practice Nurse.
7. All nurses should participate in quality initiatives to improve palliative care.
8. Specialty hospice and palliative nurses should promote continuity in palliative care across health settings and promote hospice as an option.

Domain 2: Physical Aspects of Care

1. All nurses should assess pain, dyspnea, and function, using appropriate and consistent tools in patients with serious, life-threatening illness.
2. All nurses should document findings in their care plan.
3. All nurses should follow evidence-based treatment pathways to manage pain and symptoms to reassess as appropriate.

Domain 3: Psychological and Psychiatric Aspects of Care

1. All nurses should assess depression, anxiety, and delirium, using appropriate and consistent tools in patients with serious, life-threatening illness.
2. All nurses should document findings in their care plan.
3. All nurses should follow evidence-based treatment pathways to manage psychological symptoms to reassess as appropriate.

Box 1.2 (Continued)

4. Specialty hospice and palliative nurses should assess patient and family coping and assist in developing a bereavement plan.

5. Specialty hospice and palliative nurses should participate in the development of structured bereavement programs for palliative care services.

Domain 4: Social Aspects of Care

1. All nurses should review social supports and concerns of patients and family with advanced, serious, or life-threatening illness.

2. Specialty hospice and palliative nurses should assist in development of a comprehensive social care plan that addresses the social, practical, and legal needs of the patients and caregivers, including but not limited to relationships, communication, existing social and cultural networks, decision-making, work and school settings, finances, sexuality and intimacy, caregiver availability and stress, and access to medicines and equipment.

Domain 5: Spiritual, Religious, and Existential Aspects of Care

1. Specialty hospice and palliative nurses should perform a spiritual assessment that includes religious, spiritual, and existential concerns using a structured instrument and integrate the information obtained from the assessment into the palliative care plan.

2. All nurses should refer patients and families with serious and life-threatening illness to spiritual counselors, chaplains, social community leaders, and religious leaders, as appropriate.

Domain 6: Cultural Aspects of Care

1. All nurses should assist in a cultural assessment as a component of comprehensive palliative and hospice care assessment, including, but not limited to, locus of decision-making, preferences regarding disclosure of information, truth telling and decision-making, dietary preferences, language, family communication, desire for support measures such as palliative therapies and complementary and alternative medicine, perspectives on death, suffering and grieving, and funeral and burial rituals.

Domain 7: Care of the Patient at the End of Life

1. Specialty hospice and palliative nurses should recognize and review signs and symptoms of dying with the patient, family, and staff. These discussions should be documented.

2. All nurses should assure comfort by treating symptoms for patients at the end of life (e.g., pain, dyspnea, mouth care, skin).

3. All nurses should review any cultural, religious, or pertinent rituals regarding death and after-death care with the patient and family.

(continued)

Box 1.2 (Continued)

4. All nurses should provide post-death support to the family.
5. All nurses should treat the body after death with respect, according to the cultural and religious practices of the family and in accordance with local law.

Domain 8: Ethical and Legal Aspects of Care

1. All nurses should promote and review advance care planning and appropriate documents.
2. All nurses should provide ethical care and work with an ethics committee to develop guidelines to resolve ethical dilemmas.
3. Specialty hospice and palliative nurses should understand the legal aspects of palliative care and seek legal counsel, as necessary.

guidelines be updated and kept in accordance with the NQF preferred practices. Moreover, many stakeholders inquired how the conceptual ideas of the clinical guidelines could be implemented into practice.[3] As part of the commitment to reflect changes in palliative care, healthcare policy, and healthcare research, the guidelines were updated by the four organizational members of the Hospice and Palliative Care Coalition under which the NCP was structured. Coalition organizations included the American Academy of Hospice and Palliative Medicine (AAHPM), Center to Advance Palliative Care (CAPC), Hospice and Palliative Nurses Association (HPNA), and National Hospice and Palliative Care Organization (NHPCO).

Within the review process, it was necessary to be certain that all 38 of the NQF preferred practices were reflected within the domains. To broaden the scope of the document, appraisal and discussion were undertaken within special-interest focus groups related to palliative care (i.e., pediatrics, social work, oncology, geriatrics).[3] In addition, an updated literature search was performed. To ensure the inclusivity and expansiveness of the guidelines to all settings in which palliative care is provided, clarifications were made and sections further developed. The guidelines were released again at the Annual Assembly of the AAHPM and HPNA.

From 2009 to 2013, significant maturation within the field of palliative care occurred. Palliative medicine was recognized by the American Board of Medical Specialties, thereby acknowledging palliative medicine as a distinct and well-defined field of medical practice. The number of hospice and palliative care programs across the nation with increased representation across healthcare systems and settings grew extensively. Other major developments occurred in the healthcare panorama as well. Healthcare reform within the Patient Protection and Affordable Care Act of 2010 included critical elements of palliative care.[4] A palliative care quality measurement strategy was created within the NQF, whereby new quality measures were endorsed and measurement development was enhanced.[5,6] The Joint Commission initiated Advanced Palliative Care Certification in 2011.[7] Finally, published research revealed that early-intervention palliative care had demonstrated improved quality of life, decreased psychological symptoms, and perhaps increased survival.[8,9] The NCP guidelines again were updated to reflect the field by a consortium of six key national palliative care organizations: AAHPM, CAPC, HPNA, National Association of Social Workers, NHPCO, and National Palliative Care Research Center.

Definition of Palliative Care

In the original edition, the NCP created a definition of palliative care. However, in subsequent editions, to promote consistency, the NCP chose to adopt the palliative care definition used by both the Centers for Medicare and Medicaid Services and the Federal Register, which states:

> Palliative care means patient and family-centered care that optimizes quality of life by anticipating, preventing, and treating suffering. Palliative care throughout the continuum of illness involves addressing physical, intellectual, emotional, social, and spiritual needs and to facilitate patient autonomy, access to information, and choice.[3]

In addition, the NCP described several underlying palliative care tenets:

1. Palliative care is patient- and family-centered care.
2. There is comprehensive palliative care with continuity across health settings.
3. Early introduction of palliative care concepts should begin at diagnosis of a serious or life-threatening illness by the primary team. Specialist consultation may be offered as well.
4. Palliative care may be offered concurrently with, or independent of, curative or life-prolonging care. Patient and family hopes for peace and dignity are supported throughout the course of illness, during the dying process, and after death.
5. Palliative care is interdisciplinary and collaborative. Patients, families, palliative care specialists, and other healthcare providers collaborate and communicate about care needs.
6. Palliative care team members have clinical and communication expertise.
7. The goal of palliative care is the relief of physical, psychological, emotional, and spiritual suffering of patients and families.
8. Palliative care should focus on quality care.
9. There should be equitable access to palliative care services.[3]

Eight Domains of the Guidelines for Quality Palliative Care

The NCP's guidelines included eight domains:

1. *Structure and Process of Care.* This domain addresses the organization of specialty palliative care teams and the necessary processes and

procedures for quality care delivery. The criteria emphasize coordinated assessment and continuity of care across healthcare settings. In particular, the interdisciplinary team composition, team member qualifications, and necessary education, training, and support are described. There is attention and emphasis on interdisciplinary team (IDT) engagement and collaboration with patients and families. Finally, the domain incorporates the new mandates for quality under the Patient Protection and Affordable Care Act.[3]

2. *Physical Aspects of Care.* This domain recognizes the multidimensional management of symptoms with pharmacologic, interventional, behavioral, and complementary interventions. Emphasis is placed on the assessment and treatment of physical symptoms using appropriate, validated tools. Finally, recommendations are made for the use of explicit policies in the treatment of pain and symptom management, as well as the safe prescription of controlled medications.[3]

3. *Psychological and Psychiatric Aspects of Care.* This domain acknowledges the psychological and psychiatric dimensions of palliative care. It reviews the collaborative assessment process of these diagnoses, similar to the multidimensional approach for physical aspects. It defines essential elements, including patient-family communication on assessment, diagnosis, and treatment options in the context of patient and family goals of care. Most significant, this domain now includes required criteria for a bereavement program.[3]

4. *Social Aspects of Care.* This domain emphasizes interdisciplinary engagement and collaboration with patients and families to identify, support, and capitalize on patient and family strengths. It defines essential elements of a palliative care social assessment. Notably, it includes the description of the role of the bachelor's or master's degree–prepared social work professional.[3]

5. *Spiritual, Religious, and Existential Aspects of Care.* This domain has evolved to include a spirituality definition. While simultaneously stressing interdisciplinary responsibility and collaboration in assessment and management of spiritual issues and concerns, it emphasizes the use of an appropriately trained chaplain. Requirements for staff training and education in spiritual care are described. Finally, the domain promotes spiritual and religious rituals and practices for comfort and relief.[3]

6. *Cultural Aspects of Care.* The development of this domain now includes a definition of required interdisciplinary team culture and cultural competence, highlighting culture as a source of resilience and strength for the patient and family. Cultural and linguistic competence with respect to language, literacy, and linguistically appropriate service delivery are stressed.[3]

7. *Care of the Patient at the End of Life.* The title of this domain has been changed from "Care of the Imminently Dying" to broaden care to advanced stages of illness through death. In particular, it emphasizes the

social, spiritual, and cultural aspects of care, as well as guidance to family, throughout the dying trajectory. It underscores the importance of meticulous assessment and management of pain and other symptoms. Communication, information, and documentation of the signs and symptoms of the dying process, inclusive of the patient, the family, and all other involved health providers, are underscored.[3]

8. *Ethical and Legal Aspects of Care.* This domain is separated into three sections: advance care planning, ethics, and the legal aspects of care. The responsibility of the palliative care team to promote ongoing goals of care discussions, accompanied by completion and documentation of advance care planning, is emphasized. Significant are the affirmation and acknowledgement of the frequency and complexity of palliative care ethical and legal issues. Consultation from ethics committees and legal counsel are stressed, as are team competencies in ethical principles and education regarding particular legal aspects of care. Team members' understanding of the respective scope of practice issues is emphasized.[3]

Implications of the Guidelines for Nursing

Nursing and palliative care are intertwined. Recognizing specialty palliative nursing expertise and assuring the quality of palliative nursing practice are essential to quality palliative care. The 2011 Institute of Medicine Report, *The Future of Nursing—Leading Change, Advancing Health,*[10] acknowledged the essential contributions of nursing at the bedside and in healthcare redesign, in its four messages:

1. Nurses should practice to the full extent of their education and training.
2. Nurses should achieve higher levels of education and training through an improved education system that promote seamless academic progression.
3. Nurses should be full partners, with physicians and other healthcare professionals, in redesigning healthcare in the United States.
4. Effective workforce planning and policy making require better data collection and information restructure.[10]

The NCP promotes these messages and delineates quality in three areas particularly appropriate for nursing and consistent with the Institute of Medicine report: professional development, education, and certification. Nurses at all levels can promote consistent roles, job descriptions, and education. The NCP guidelines provide nationally recognized definitions of hospice and palliative care, acknowledging the role of nursing in the IDT and care coordination and thereby promoting practice to the full extent of nurses' education and training. Because participating NCP members include representation from nursing, hospice, research, palliative care, and social work, the guidelines were meant to be inclusive across all settings. The NCP guidelines establish essential elements of specialist palliative care that promote quality, consistency, and reliability of services. This helps distinguish between primary palliative nursing and specialty palliative nursing.

Perhaps this will also promote nurses' achievement of higher education and training in academic programs with palliative care.

Moreover, because the NCP guidelines are meant to guide program development and benchmarking, they can assist palliative nurse leaders or coordinators in program development. The NCP guidelines may promote more effective data collection and information-gathering by nurses. As nationally recognized guidelines, they can be incorporated easily into a program. Finally, they allow the palliative care nurses to measure their programs in terms of quality and breadth. Box 1.2 offers an overview of how the guidelines can be implemented for nurses.

Adoption of the Guidelines by Nurses

There are many important reasons for nurses to adopt the *Clinical Practice Guidelines*. They offer a framework to care, educational areas, and criteria for benchmarking. Nurses practice in a variety of settings that may have palliative care programs. These include acute care programs, ambulatory care programs, rehabilitation facility programs, community programs, home care programs, hospice programs, long-term care facilities, accountable care organizations, and patient medical homes. As a framework to care, the NCP guidelines assist nurses in creating quality palliative services or developing quality programs in all of these settings. In particular, the structure for bereavement can promote essential program components in the various domains (e.g., quality improvement processes, bereavement programs, spiritual care, and cultural care). The emphasis on consistency is important, particularly in orientation, job descriptions, and peer review. Assisting programs in developing critical organizational structures and processes may lead to improved staff retention and morale.

As an education tool, the guidelines offer the content for programs and can promote more effective educational programs. The scope of potential topics includes the focus of orientation, communication, pain and symptom assessment, social-cultural assessment, and spiritual assessment. These areas are important to nurses in all settings. Moreover, the guidelines support the use of research and evidence-based practice. Just as important, the essential aspects of ethical foundations and legal regulations assist nurses in scope-of-practice issues and mitigate moral distress by having more clearly delineated processes for conflict resolution.

As benchmarks, the NCP guidelines assist nurses and palliative care programs in achieving the highest possible quality of care in all health settings by ensuring adherence to the highest standards of care. Their use may result in improved patient outcomes and better compliance with state and federal regulations. Because appropriate resource utilization is a common concern, the emphasis on community assessment and communication across settings and specialties may provide a nursing benchmark. Moreover, the strict descriptions of pain and symptom assessment, management, use of assessment tools, and evidence-based practice are significant. These criteria may help with improved patient and family satisfaction in pain and symptom control. Moreover, domain 2, Physical Aspects of Care, and domain 3, Psychological and Psychiatric Aspects of Care, may help organizations meet evidence requirements for Magnet status in the following areas: Structural Empowerment concerning nursing image and professional development; Exemplary Professional Practice concerning consultation and resources, autonomy, and interdisciplinary relationships; New Knowledge, Innovation, and Improvements concerning quality improvement; and Empirical Quality Results concerning quality of care.[11] They can also facilitate accreditation by The Joint Commission in the areas of pain management, culturally competent care, and end of life care.

Conclusion

The NCP *Clinical Practice Guidelines for Quality Palliative Care* are a significant resource, offering nurses a framework for quality care in all settings. The guidelines are appropriate for a range of populations, including neonates, children, adults, and older adults; a range of chronic progressive and serious life-threatening illnesses, injuries, and trauma; and a range of vulnerable and under-resourced populations (e.g., homeless individuals, immigrants, individuals with low income, oppressed racial and ethnic groups, veterans, prisoners, older adults, and individuals with mental illness). Finally, they are appropriate for any setting because they facilitate partnerships in caring for patients with debilitating and life-limiting illnesses and offer support for nurses in delivering care, particularly for long-term patients.

References

1. National Consensus Project for Quality Palliative Care. *Clinical Practice Guidelines for Quality Palliative Care*. Pittsburgh, PA: National Consensus Project for Quality Palliative Care; 2004.

2. National Quality Forum. *A National Framework and Preferred Practices for Palliative and Hospice Care Quality: A Consensus Report*. Washington, DC: National Quality Forum; 2006.

3. National Consensus Project for Quality Palliative Care. *Clinical Practice Guidelines for Quality Palliative Care*. 3rd ed. Pittsburgh, PA: National Consensus Project; 2013.

4. Patient Protection and Affordable Care Act (PPACA), Public Law 111-148, §2702, Title III (B)(III) Section 3140, 124, Stat. 119, 318-319, Consolidating amendments made by Title X of the Act and the Health Care and Education Reconciliation Act of 2010. Washington, DC: 2010. http://www.gpo.gov/fdsys/pkg/PLAW-111publ148/html/PLAW-111publ148.htm. Last updated March 10, 2010. Accessed October 1, 2014.

5. National Quality Forum. *Palliative Care and End of Life Care: A Consensus Report*. Washington, DC: National Quality Forum; 2012. http://www.qualityforum.org/Publications/2012/04/Palliative_Care_and_End of Life_Care%E2%80%94A_Consensus_Report.aspx. Last updated August 29, 2012. Accessed October 1, 2014.

6. National Quality Forum. *Measure Applications Partnership: Performance Measurement Coordination Strategies for Hospice and Palliative Care Final Report.* Washington, DC: 2012. http://www.qualityforum.org/Publications/2012/06/Performance_Measurement_Coordination_Strategy_for_Hospice_and_Palliative_Care.aspx. Last updated February 8, 2013. Accessed October 1, 2014.

7. The Joint Commission. Advanced certification in palliative care. 2011. http://www.jointcommission.org/certification/palliative_care.aspx. Accessed October 1, 2014.

8. Bakitas M, Lyons KD, Hegel MT, et al. Effects of a palliative care intervention on clinical outcomes in patients with advanced cancer: the Project ENABLE II randomized controlled trial. *JAMA.* 2009;302(7):741–749.

9. Temel J, Greer J, Muzikansky A, et al. Early palliative care for patients with metastatic non-small cell lung cancer. *N Engl J Med.* 2010;363:733–742.

10. Institute of Medicine. *The Future of Nursing: Leading Change, Advancing Health.* Washington, DC: National Academies Press; 2011.

11. American Nurses Credentialing Center. Announcing a new model for ANCC's. Magnet Recognition Program©. 2008 *Magnet News.* http://www.nursecredentialing.org/MagnetModel.aspx#Empirical. Accessed October 1, 2014.

Chapter 2

Hospital-Based Palliative Care

Patricia Maani-Fogelman and Marie Bakitas

Hospital-based palliative care (HBPC) is the continually evolving moral imperative: the number of Americans living with chronic illness exceeds 90 million, and seven of every 10 Americans die from complications of a chronic illness.[1] This burden is significantly higher in the Medicare population, in which the majority of deaths are attributable to nine diagnoses: congestive heart failure, chronic lung disease, cancer, coronary artery disease, renal failure, peripheral vascular disease, diabetes, chronic liver disease, and dementia.[2] As the 2012 Dartmouth Atlas of Healthcare noted, "Patients with chronic illness in their last two years of life account for about 32% of total Medicare spending, much of it going toward physician and hospital fees associated with repeated hospitalizations."[3] Moving forward with better integration of palliative care in the end of life (EOL) care of inpatients, one must consider the following: What do our patients desire at the end of their life? Where do they want to spend the time they have left? Closer to home, in the hospital, or at home? When medical interventions are deemed medically inappropriate or unlikely to yield a meaningful benefit, do they want to pursue treatment or "cease and desist," with transition to a different plan of care?

When comparing location of death for Medicare beneficiaries in 2005 to 2009 versus 2000, fewer numbers died in the hospital, yet use of intensive care unit services and healthcare transitions increased most in in the last few weeks of life.[1,2]

Although research confirms that patients with advanced illness report a preference to die at home, most are still dying in the hospital. Care was rarely aligned with reported preferences: among the patients who indicated that they preferred to die at home, the majority (55%) died in the hospital. The evidence demonstrates the vital importance of high-quality delivery of palliative care services within the context of inpatient care, especially when the admission is likely to become the patient's terminal admission. This highlights the importance of pioneering methodologies for EOL care to facilitate patient and family engagement in early discussions of preferences for EOL care in advanced medical illness before the catastrophe strikes and aggressive interventions are initiated at end of life.[3,4] Chronic illness and longer life were the legacy of the 20th century. However, the healthcare system did not keep pace with medical advances. The hospital became a common location for a good portion of EOL care, despite Americans' stated preference for death at home.[4] An analysis of the experience of dying among chronically ill Medicare recipients revealed more hospice care in 2007 than in 2003. Although a percentage of seriously ill patients experienced their final admission in a critical care unit, by and large, hospital deaths occurred in non-critical care units and could have been anticipated for hours or days before death actually occurred. Despite this opportunity to provide comfort measures during the dying process, patients dying in the acute care hospital experienced pain, dyspnea, anxiety, and other distressing symptoms.[5] Hospitals were designed primarily to provide acute, episodic care to persons with acute illness, rather than comfort and continuity to persons who were not expected to survive a particular disease or episode of illness. Therefore, fundamental system reform and redesign were needed to improve (and possibly prevent) hospital care of persons with life-limiting illness. As Berwick wrote:

> Academic medicine has a major opportunity to support the redesign of healthcare systems; it ought to bear part of the burden for accelerating the pace, confidence, and pervasiveness of that change. . . . "Where is the randomized trial?" is, for many purposes, the right question, but for many others, it is the wrong question, a myopic one. A better one is broader: "What is everyone learning?" Asking the question that way will help clinicians and researchers see further in navigating toward improvement.[6]

This is a call to action, particularly for nurses, because nursing care is the primary service provided during hospital admission, and much of the care and the system that patients experience could be influenced by nurses, at all organizational levels. How nurses are learning and sharing their knowledge will further direct the process of patient care. Most other types of care, such as physician consultation, diagnostic tests, and pharmaceutical treatments, do not generally require inpatient admission.

HBPC programs have begun to change the quality and quantity of hospitalized deaths. Nurses have served as leaders and active team members to define, direct, and lead multidisciplinary and interdisciplinary teams and modify efforts at multiple levels of the hospital care system in order to improve the complex care process for persons with life-limiting illness. Improved palliative care structure, standards for care processes, and the measurement of outcomes have begun to come about as a result of the development of HBPC programs (Box 2.1). The new millennium marked the "end of the beginning" of the discipline of palliative care.

The case study of Mr. X demonstrates the importance of early palliative care intervention so that advance directives and patient- and family-centered care can be delivered. The introduction of palliative care at the time of diagnosis allowed for appropriate and effective use of the palliative care services. When the patient is identified early in the course of illness, the palliative care team can act as a resource for advance care planning, goals of care discussions, bereavement support, pain and

Box 2.1 Case Study: Mr. X

Mr. X is a 47-year-old man who was driving home from work when he swerved and lost control of his vehicle; the vehicle travelled down an embankment and crashed, and he was trapped. He was found unconscious by an oncoming driver, who called 911. Mr. X's Glasgow Coma Score was 6T, and active medical problems on admission to the intensive care and trauma unit from the motor vehicle collision included subarachnoid hemorrhage, subdural hemorrhage, multiple intraparenchymal hemorrhages, left parieto-occipital scalp laceration, and right upper lung collapse. Electroencephalogram revealed diffuse slowing consistent with encephalopathy without evidence of epileptiform activity. Magnetic resonance imaging showed diffuse widespread axonal injury to the brain with large areas of contusion and hemorrhagic transformation.

The palliative care team (PCT) was consulted on admission and was present for initial and all subsequent meetings with the patient's wife and extended family. There was noted conflict between family members with regard to the plan of care and perceptions about Mr. X's preferences. Despite aggressive interventions, Mr. X did not demonstrate neurologic improvement and continued to decline with loss of reflexive maneuvers and ventilator-dependent respiratory failure. The medical teams were in agreement that his prognosis was extremely poor and that he would not recover to a meaningful level of function. Multiple family meetings were held, and his wife shared that her husband would not desire artificial means of support in the event he was not going to make a full and meaningful recovery to independent function (preadmission baseline.) His parents and siblings felt that everything should be continued and escalated and that life in a nursing home was still better than death. His adult children were conflicted, feeling caught in the struggle between angry grandparents and their mother.

During a family meeting on hospital day 5, the patient's father and brother asked when Mr. X would recover to return home. The PCT reviewed with the family that because of the devastating extent of the injuries, he would require continuous custodial care in a skilled facility and he would not regain any independent function. His siblings then replied that would not be an acceptable life for the patient, who was an outdoor enthusiast and enjoyed a very active lifestyle. His parents also agreed with this assessment. His wife and children were in agreement as well. The PCT reviewed the options for Mr. X's plan of care with his spouse and extended family. The family decided to elect terminal extubation and transition to comfort measures and inquired about how his comfort would be assured. What parameters do you assess for comfort? How do you assess them?

After the meeting, the family asked for immediate extubation with transition to comfort care. The PCT assisted with terminal extubation orders, and the comfort measures order set was started. The patient

(continued)

Box 2.1 (Continued)

was medicated before extubation and placed on an opioid infusion to ensure that he remained free of respiratory distress and pain. After extubation, the critical care nurses assisted with personal care and removed all nonessential medical equipment (i.e., ventilator, infusion devices, code cart) from the patient's room to allow more room for family to remain with patient. The family returned to the room and remained with the patient until his death.

symptom management, and psychosocial issues. As the patient nears death, and the goal of care becomes focused more on comfort, the palliative care team will be a familiar part of the care team during a potentially stressful time.

Quality of Care Issues Identified in This Case

- The patient was identified early in the trajectory of illness.
- Patient and family values and preferences for care were identified early and integrated into the plan of care.
- A team approach allowed for various members to assist with the patient's diverse needs across the entire episode of illness.
- Palliative care involvement occurred in the hospital setting. Continuity occurred across all settings.
- The patient's preference for location of death was met.

Brief History and Definitions of Hospital-Based Palliative Care

In 1974, the Royal Victoria Hospital in Montreal, Canada, developed one of the first initiatives in North America to improve HBPC. They developed a palliative care service to meet the needs of hospitalized patients who were terminally ill within the general hospital setting.[7] The palliative care service was an integral part of the Royal Victoria Hospital and included a 1,000-bed teaching hospital affiliated with McGill University, consisting of five complementary clinical components: (1) the Palliative Care Unit, (2) the home care service, (3) the consultation team, (4) the palliative care clinic, and (5) the bereavement follow-up program. Members of an interdisciplinary team were involved with the care of these patients, and the focus was on holistic care with pain control and symptom management.

Three decades later, these basic palliative care concepts are becoming more prevalent in many U.S. hospitals. In the United States, a number of milestones over the past four decades have shaped the evolution of care of the seriously ill. In the 1970s, the concept of home-based hospice programs (often volunteer only) migrated to the United States from Europe and Canada. Since that time, a number of professional, medical, societal, and academic endeavors have coalesced in the form of HBPC programs. HBPC adapts and "upstreams" many of the principles of hospice care into mainstream medicine. Although there is no requirement for all healthcare systems to have such a program, palliative care is gradually being recognized as a "standard of care." Some key goals of HBPC are (1) to improve clinical quality of care for seriously ill patients; (2) to increase patient and family satisfaction with care; (3) to meet the demand of a growing, chronically ill, elderly demographic; (4) to serve as "classrooms" for the next generation of clinicians who need to provide better care to the seriously ill; and (5) to provide value-added, cost-effective care in the face of a national healthcare and economic crisis.[8]

Although many of the data to support the evolution of HBPC have come from care deficits identified in hospitalized patients at the very end of life, the goal of HBPC is to improve the quality of life of persons with life-limiting illness much earlier in the course of illness, across all settings of healthcare.

A number of definitions of HBPC exist, but they contain similar elements. In 1990, the World Health Organization defined palliative care as care that "seeks to address not only physical pain, but also emotional, social, and spiritual pain to achieve the best possible quality of life for patients and their families. Palliative care extends the principles of hospice care to a broader population that could benefit from receiving this type of care earlier in their illness or disease process."[9] An HBPC program has been defined by the American Hospital Association as "an organized program providing specialized medical care, drugs, or therapies for the management of acute or chronic pain and/or the control of symptoms administered by specially trained physicians and other clinicians; and supportive care services, such as counseling on advance directives, spiritual care, and social services, to patients with advanced disease and their families."[8] The Center to Advance Palliative Care (CAPC) defines HBPC as "an interdisciplinary medical team focused on symptom management, intensive patient–physician–family communication, clarifying goals of treatment and coordination of care across healthcare settings."[10] In Temel's (2010) landmark study, "Early Palliative Care for Patients with Metastatic Non–Small-Cell Lung Cancer,"[11] lung cancer patients who received palliative care along with conventional treatment survived 2.7 months longer than patients who received only standard oncologic care! Published by the *New England Journal of Medicine,* this study clearly demonstrated the value, need, and importance of palliative medicine interventions for patients with advanced, life-limiting illness.

The good news is that since the American Hospital Association survey began to measure the availability of HBPC programs in 2000, there has been a steady growth. This positive movement is tempered by two issues. First, there is wide variability in patients' access to palliative care programs across the United States. In particular, the southern region of the United States at 41% has the lowest availability of programs. Second, despite definitions of HBPC, mandatory standards of care as yet do not exist; therefore, programs can vary in their quality, components, and emphasis on the missions of service, research, and education.[12]

Primary, Secondary, and Tertiary Models of Hospital-Based Palliative Care

Promoting HBPC requires a myriad of resources. Depending on the model of palliative care being introduced, the required resources can vary greatly. For example, some changes may require financial support through construction or addition of staff, whereas other changes are less resource-intensive. Regardless of the healthcare system and the availability of resources, all healthcare practitioners have the ability to introduce palliative care concepts and use already established resources to develop or improve their palliative care services. Institutions with limited resources may choose a primary model that focuses on enhancing existing services and clinician education, whereas secondary and tertiary palliative care programs may provide multiple services, including inpatient and/or outpatient consult teams, an inpatient palliative care or hospice unit, and a home-care program, all under the jurisdiction of a single hospital system. A full-service approach can ease transitions among different levels of care and has the potential to provide optimal seamless palliative care. CAPC also offers various consensus guidelines for operational and inpatient unit metrics that hospitals can use to measure programs for quality, sustainability, and growth[12] (Table 2.1).

Primary Palliative Care

Primary palliative care should be available at all hospitals. This level of care requires, at a minimum, clinician education in the basics of pain and symptom management. Primary palliative care refers to a level of care whereby basic skills and competencies are required of all physicians, nurses, and other healthcare practitioners who come in contact with persons with life-limiting illness. The National Consensus Project (NCP), the National Quality Forum (NQF), and The Joint Commission (TJC) have each

Table 2.1 Metric Categories	
Metric Domain	**Examples**
Operational	Patient demographics (diagnosis, age, gender, ethnicity), referring clinician, disposition, hospital length of stay
Clinical	Symptom scores, psychosocial symptom assessment
Customer (patient, family, referring clinicians)	Patient, family, referring clinician satisfaction surveys
Financial	Costs (pre- and post-HBPC consultation), inpatient palliative unit, net loss/gain for inpatient deaths

HBPC, hospital-based palliative care.

Source: Data from Weissman DE, Meier DE, Spragens LH. Center to Advance Palliative Care. palliative care consultation service metrics: consensus recommendations. *J Palliat Med.* 2008;11(10):1294–1298.

identified standards that should be addressed in all hospitals and other settings (see later discussion). All practitioners should be competent at this level.

Clinicians can gain the knowledge, attitudes, and skills needed to provide palliative care to their patients through basic palliative care training and clinical practice. There is a growing availability of continuing education, including established formal programs for all disciplines to improve their knowledge of basic palliative care principles. The End of Life Nursing Education Consortium (ELNEC) and Education for Physicians on End of Life Care (EPEC) are two comprehensive educational programs that can provide such information.

Secondary Palliative Care

Secondary palliative care refers to a model in which all providers have a minimum level of competence and, in addition, have specialists who provide palliative care through an interdisciplinary team (IDT), specialized unit, or both. The development and success of these specialized services will come about as a result of strong leadership, marketing, and accessibility.[13] It is not necessary for an IDT or unit to evaluate every patient with palliative care needs who is admitted to the hospital, but these specially trained clinicians are available as a resource and guide for their colleagues.

Tertiary Palliative Care

Teaching hospitals and academic centers with teams of experts in palliative care are classified as tertiary organizations. A tertiary-level program may serve as a consultant to primary- and secondary-level practices in difficult clinical situations or as a model program to assist developing centers.[14] These centers also serve as training programs for incoming palliative medicine providers, with fellowship programs ranging from one to two years for both physicians and nurses. Practitioners and institutions involved at the tertiary level of palliative care are also involved in educational and research activities.[15] Multidisciplinary training programs for nurses and physicians are an important function of a tertiary center (see later discussion). Tertiary centers also have an obligation to perform research to enhance the evidence base for palliative care.

It is the responsibility of all hospitals and healthcare organizations to be competent, at a minimum, at the primary level of palliative care. Organizations at different levels may choose among different components of care to incorporate into their model. Some components are less resource-intense (e.g., staff education, care pathways), whereas others may require additional allocations of budget and personnel. The latter resources include IDTs, specialized palliative care units (PCUs), outpatient or ambulatory palliative care clinics, and structured outreach or strong relationships with skilled nursing facilities and home-based hospice programs.

Inpatient Interdisciplinary Consult Team

A growing literature summarizes the development of palliative care consultation teams within hospitals to offer specialized consultation and expertise to patients, families, and other healthcare providers.[16,17] Dunlop and

Hockley published a manual in 1990, and a second edition in 1998, describing the experience in England.[18] They described the movement as one that tries to take the hospice philosophy of care and bring it into the hospital, using a consultancy team. A number of U.S. and European hospital-based teams have described their experiences. Among the components of successful teams are an interdisciplinary approach, physician and nonphysician referral, rapid response to requested consultations, around-the-clock availability, and ability to follow patients through all care settings.

IDTs can be effective in modeling behaviors that are supportive of appropriate HBPC, but they should also recommend infrastructure and organizational changes as part of their approach to consultation. Gathering data about demographic statistics on the location and nature of regular consultations may help to identify the need for particular institutional policies and procedures. For example, if a particular unit or care provider has difficulty managing patients with dyspnea on a regular basis, targeted educational approaches and treatment algorithms or standardized orders may help achieve consistent and long-lasting change. Theoretically, an IDT could "put itself out of business" with such an approach. Conversely, teams may become "stretched too thin" in their attempts to meet the needs of their organization; however, the news remains positive: to-date, teams have not reported the need to dissolve as an outcome of implementing system changes.

Studies have begun to examine the impact of IDTs on the overall care of hospitalized, seriously ill patients.[19] However, this is challenging research, and as in any multicomponent intervention, it is difficult to identify exactly which components or processes of the team are responsible for the outcomes. Valid, reliable measures and multimethod research are likely to be needed to capture this information. Maintaining an IDT can be costly; therefore, it is imperative to continue to evaluate programs and strengthen the evidence base to provide economic justification for many hospitals. A consensus panel has recommended minimum data that should be collected by all consultation services.[19]

Inpatient Hospice and Palliative Care Units
Some hospitals, faced with the problem of providing high-quality palliative care, have found the development of a specialized unit to be the solution. U.S. hospitals have varying amounts of experience with opening specialized units for the care of patients with hospice or palliative care needs.[20,21] An inpatient unit has some advantages and disadvantages. Advantages include:

- Patients requiring palliative care have a familiar place to go during the exacerbations and remissions that come with progressive disease.
- Unit staff and policies are under the control and financing of experts trained as a team who are skillful at difficult care and communications.
- Patients may get palliative care earlier, if other care teams see the advantages of this approach and trust that patients will receive good care.

Providers who monitor their patients on these units (if allowed) can learn valuable lessons about palliative care that can be carried forward to future patients. These future patients may not require admission to the PCU for some types of care. Some disadvantages of creating a PCU include:

- It can prevent others from learning valuable palliative care techniques, if the PCU staff is seen as "specialized" and is secluded in one area.
- Care providers may come to rely on this expertise instead of learning palliative care techniques themselves.
- If PCU transfer includes a transfer of doctors to a palliative care specialist, patients and families may feel abandoned by their primary team in the final hours.
- Hospice providers fear loss of the hospice philosophy when a PCU exists in the context of the general hospital.

Outpatient or Ambulatory Palliative Care Clinics

In an ideal world, patients with life-limiting illness spend most of their time outside of the hospital, with only occasional need for attention by a palliative care specialist. Transitions of care are a common area of difficulty for patients with palliative care needs. An outpatient service can serve as an initial point of referral for patients early in their disease process,[22] or it may allow a discharged patient to continue to have specialized management of their symptoms and other needs. A number of models of delivering outpatient care exist,[21,22] including a consultative model in which palliative care clinicians participate in other disease-focused outpatient visits (e.g., in clinics serving patients with advanced lung disease, congestive heart failure, cancer, or amyotrophic lateral sclerosis) to geographic space allotted only to palliative care clinicians and patients. Outpatient services are still considered a novel, less frequent service component of HBPC in most organizations; however, this has become a recognized service delivery need that is quickly growing, in demand and popularity, across national health systems today.

Liaisons with Skilled Nursing Facilities and Home Hospice

Perhaps one of the most important ways to improve HBPC is to develop strong relationships with other healthcare agencies outside of the hospital so that alternatives to inpatient admission for palliative care exist. Alternatives such as home hospice care or skilled hospice care within assisted-living centers, freestanding hospices, or specially designated areas in nursing homes or rehabilitation facilities, can provide expert palliative and hospice care. However, some areas of the United States lack these options. For example, in some rural areas, healthcare services, such as visiting nurse agencies, home care, hospice, and skilled nursing facilities, are sparse, or staff may feel unprepared to care for people who require intensive palliative care. Some visiting nurse and home care agencies may see so few symptomatic, seriously ill patients that it is difficult for staff to maintain adequate palliative care and hospice expertise in these agencies. There continues to be a need to develop models and strengthen relationships between HBPC programs and community agencies that will provide palliative care services, before or after hospital palliative care services. An area for further growth and exploration is the branching out of palliative care delivery to satellite locations, with advanced illness patients, such as those with end-stage renal disease or class III or IV heart failure, and nursing home residents with multiple advanced and complex comorbid medical conditions.

Bereavement Services

Improving HBPC does not end with the development of mechanisms to ensure peaceful, pain-free patient death. Although accomplishing this goal is surely a comfort to family and friends, bereavement care for survivors is an important final step in the process of HBPC. Which families are most in need of specific services? Identifying families at the greatest risk has been the topic of palliative care research, particularly in evaluating the quality of palliative care services.

Bereavement services for survivors are an important part of the total care plan, after the patient's death. NQF preferred practices standard for bereavement care indicates organizations should: "Facilitate effective grieving by implementing in a timely manner a bereavement care plan after the patient's death, when the family remains the focus of care."[23] Adverse physical and psychological outcomes of unsupported grief are known to occur during the bereavement period. Because of this, bereavement services are a typical component of the services offered to families when patients die as part of a hospice program. Because not all deaths in the United States have hospice involvement, a large portion of families must rely on bereavement follow-up offered by other care providers. Although historically, few hospitals routinely offered bereavement services to families after patients died in the hospital, a growing interest in such programs has come about as a result of implementing HBPC programs.

Bereavement services can address currently unmet needs of survivors, who can benefit from resources that offer information and support on coping with the loss. Having follow-up contact with decedents' family members can also provide HBPC programs with information about the effectiveness of EOL care. Families' perspectives should be sought about what went well and what could be improved. For example, results of a focus group of bereaved family members indicated that, although the family was quite satisfied with pain management, breathing changes and dyspnea were not anticipated and were very distressing. Hence, this became a target for improving EOL care in one hospital.

Use of family proxy perspectives is an emerging area of research and quality improvement. Press-Ganey, a healthcare measurement and improvement company that is well known for collecting patient satisfaction data after hospital discharge, now also has a survey to collect family perspectives on the EOL experience in the hospital. This survey asks about topics such as care at the time of death; care provided by nurses, physicians, chaplains, social workers, and others; environment; family care; symptoms; and overall satisfaction with care.

Standardized bereavement care can take many forms and can result in improved family satisfaction with care. These actions might include sending a sympathy note or establishing some other contact from a staff member, mailing a list of local bereavement resources or a pamphlet, and delaying the time before a hospital bill is mailed out to prevent its coinciding with funeral or memorial services. A variety of bereavement services have been developed for parents that specifically address their needs after the death of an infant or child.

The Joint Commission

TJC is one of the paramount accreditation organizations for hospitals and other healthcare organizations. The purpose of TJC is to continuously improve the safety and quality of care provided to the public. TJC is an independent, not-for-profit organization, and perhaps its most important benefit is that TJC-accredited organizations make a commitment to continuous improvement in patient care. During an accreditation survey, TJC evaluates a group's performance by using a set of standards that cross eight functional areas: (1) rights, responsibilities, and ethics; (2) continuum of care; (3) education and communication; (4) health promotion and disease prevention; (5) leadership; (6) management of human resources; (7) management of information; and (8) improving network performance.[24]

In 2004, a specific palliative care focus was introduced within two standards: (1) rights, responsibilities, and ethics; and (2) the provision of care, treatment, and services. The goal of the rights, responsibilities, and ethics standard is to improve outcomes by recognizing and respecting the rights of each patient and working in an ethical manner. Care, treatment, and services are to be provided in a way that respects the person and fosters dignity. The performance standard states that a patient's family should be involved in the care, treatment, and services, if the patient desires. Care, treatment, and services are provided through ongoing assessments of care, meeting the patient's needs, and either successfully discharging the patient or providing referral or transfer of the patient for continuing care.[24] More detailed information is available by contacting TJC or visiting its website at http://www.jcrinc.com.

These standards incorporated a stronger emphasis on palliative care practices within organizations. Hence, organizations are being held accountable for the manner in which they provide appropriate palliative care. It is in the public's best interest that TJC requires organizations to adhere to these provisions for a successful accreditation. In 2008, a process to develop specific "Certification for Palliative Care Programs" was begun, and in 2011, TJC's *Advanced Certification Program for Palliative Care* was launched. The standards for palliative care certification are built on the NCP's *Clinical Practice Guidelines for Quality Palliative Care* (Table 2.2) and the NQF's *National Framework and Preferred Practices for Palliative and Hospice Care Quality* (Table 2.3). Standards and expectations were developed using

Table 2.2 National Quality Forum Preferred Practices Organized by National Consensus Project: Domains of Quality Palliative Care

National Consensus Project Domains of Quality Palliative Care	National Quality Forum Preferred Practices*
1. Structure and processes of care	1. Provide palliative and hospice care by an interdisciplinary team of skilled palliative care professionals, including, for example, physicians, nurses, social workers, pharmacists, spiritual care counselors, and others who collaborate with primary healthcare professional(s). **[4. STAFFING]**
	2. Provide access to palliative and hospice care that is responsive to the patient and family, 24 hours a day, seven days a week. **[3. AVAILABILITY]**
	3. Provide continuing education to all healthcare professionals on the domains of palliative care and hospice care. **[8. EDUCATION]**
	4. Provide adequate training and clinical support to ensure that professional staff is confident in their ability to provide palliative care for patients. **[12. STAFF WELLNESS]**
	5. Hospice care and specialized palliative care professionals should be appropriately trained, credentialed, and/or certified in their area of expertise. **[4. STAFFING]**
	6. Formulate, utilize, and regularly review a timely care plan based on a comprehensive interdisciplinary assessment of the values, preferences, goals, and needs of the patient and family and, to the extent that privacy laws permit, ensure that the plan is broadly disseminated, both internally and externally, to all professionals involved in the patient's care.
	7. Ensure that upon transfer between healthcare settings, there is timely and thorough communication of the patient's goals, preferences, values, and clinical information so that continuity of care and seamless follow-up are assured. **[11. CONTINUITY OF CARE]**
	8. Healthcare professionals should present hospice as an option to all patients and families when death within a year would not be surprising and should reintroduce the hospice option as the patient declines. **[11. CONTINUITY OF CARE]**
	9. Patients and caregivers should be asked by palliative and hospice care programs to assess physicians'/healthcare professionals' ability to discuss hospice as an option.

(continued)

Table 2.2 (Continued)

National Consensus Project Domains of Quality Palliative Care	National Quality Forum Preferred Practices*
	10. Enable patients to make informed decisions about their care by educating them on the process of their disease, prognosis, and benefits and burdens of potential interventions.
	11. Provide education and support to families and unlicensed caregivers based on the patient's individualized care plan to ensure safe and appropriate care for the patient.
2. Physical aspects of care	12. Measure and document pain, dyspnea, constipation, and other symptoms using available standardized scales. **[5. MEASUREMENT; 6. QI]**
	13. Assess and manage symptoms and side effects in a timely, safe, and effective manner to a level that is acceptable to the patient and family. **[5. MEASUREMENT; 6. QI]**
3. Psychological and psychiatric aspects of care	14. Measure and document anxiety, depression, delirium, behavioral disturbances, and other common psychological symptoms using available standardized scales. **[5. MEASUREMENT; 6. QI]**
	15. Manage anxiety, depression, delirium, behavioral disturbances, and other common psychological symptoms in a timely, safe, and effective manner to a level that is acceptable to the patient and family. **[5. MEASUREMENT; 6. QI]**
	16. Assess and manage the psychological reactions of patients and families (including stress, anticipatory grief, and coping) in a regular, ongoing fashion in order to address emotional and functional impairment and loss. **[5. MEASUREMENT; 6. QI]**
	17. Develop and offer a grief and bereavement care plan to provide services to patients and families before and for at least 13 months after the death of the patient. **[9. BEREAVEMENT]**
4. Social aspects of care	18. Conduct regular patient and family care conferences with physicians and other appropriate members of the interdisciplinary team to provide information, to discuss goals of care, disease prognosis, and advance care planning, and to offer support.

(continued)

25

Table 2.2 (Continued)

National Consensus Project Domains of Quality Palliative Care	National Quality Forum Preferred Practices*
	19. Develop and implement a comprehensive social care plan that addresses the social, practical, and legal needs of the patient and caregivers, including, but not limited to, relationships, communication, existing social and cultural networks, decision-making, work and school settings, finances, sexuality and intimacy, caregiver availability and stress, and access to medicines and equipment. **[4. STAFFING]**
5. Spiritual, religious, and existential aspects of care	20. Develop and document a plan based on an assessment of religious, spiritual, and existential concerns using a structured instrument and integrate the information obtained from the assessment into the palliative care plan. **[4. STAFFING]**
	21. Provide information about the availability of spiritual care services and make spiritual care available, either through organizational spiritual care counseling or through the patient's own clergy relationships. **[4. STAFFING]**
	22. Specialized palliative and hospice care teams should include spiritual care professionals appropriately trained and certified in palliative care. **[4. STAFFING]**
	23. Specialized palliative and hospice spiritual care professionals should build partnerships with community clergy and provide education and counseling related to end of life care. **[4. STAFFING]**
6. Cultural aspects of care	24. Incorporate cultural assessment as a component of comprehensive palliative and hospice care assessment, including, but not limited to, locus of decision-making; preferences regarding disclosure of information; truth telling and decision-making; dietary preferences; language; family communication; desire for support measures such as palliative therapies and complementary and alternative medicine; perspectives on death, suffering, and grieving; and funeral and burial rituals.
	25. Provide professional interpreter services and culturally sensitive materials in the patient's and family's preferred language.
7. Care of the imminently dying patient	26. Recognize and document the transition to the active dying phase, and communicate to the patient, family, and staff the expectation of imminent death.

(continued)

Table 2.2 (Continued)

National Consensus Project Domains of Quality Palliative Care	National Quality Forum Preferred Practices*
	27. Educate the family on a timely basis regarding the signs and symptoms of imminent death in an age-appropriate, developmentally appropriate, and culturally appropriate manner.
	28. As part of the ongoing care planning process, routinely ascertain and document patient and family wishes about the care setting for the site of death and fulfill patient and family preferences when possible. **[11. CONTINUITY OF CARE]**
	29. Provide adequate dosage of analgesics and sedatives, as appropriate, to achieve patient comfort during the active dying phase and address concerns and fears about using narcotics and analgesics hastening death.
	30. Treat the body after death with respect according to the cultural and religious practices of the family and in accordance with local law. **[9. BEREAVEMENT]**
	31. Facilitate effective grieving by implementing, in a timely manner, a bereavement care plan after the patient's death, when the family remains the focus of care. **[9. BEREAVEMENT]**
8. Ethical and legal aspects of care	32. Document the designated surrogate or decision-maker, in accordance with state law for every patient in primary, acute, and long-term care and in palliative and hospice care.
	33. Document the patient and/or surrogate preferences for goals of care, treatment options, and setting of care at first assessment and at frequent intervals, as conditions change.
	34. Convert the patient treatment goals into medical orders and ensure that the information is transferable and applicable across care settings, including long-term care, emergency medical services, and hospital care, through a program such as the Physician Orders for Life-Sustaining Treatment (POLST) program.
	35. Make advance directives and surrogacy designations available across care settings, while protecting patient privacy and adherence to HIPAA regulations, for example, by using Internet-based registries or electronic personal health records.

(continued)

Table 2.2 (Continued)	
National Consensus Project Domains of Quality Palliative Care	**National Quality Forum Preferred Practices***
	36. Develop healthcare and community collaborations to promote advance care planning and the completion of advance directives for all individuals, for example, the Respecting Choices and Community Conversations on Compassionate Care programs.
	37. Establish or have access to ethics committees or ethics consultation across care settings to address ethical conflicts at the end of life.
	38. For minors with decision-making capacity, document the child's views and preferences for medical care, including assent for treatment, and give these preferences appropriate weight in decision-making. Make appropriate professional staff members available to both the child and the adult decision-maker for consultation and intervention, when the child's wishes differ from those of the adult decision-maker.

*[BOLDED] entries refer to corresponding domain from Weissman DE, Meier DE. Operational features for hospital palliative care programs: consensus recommendations. *J Palliat Med.* 2009;12(1):21–25.

experts in palliative care and key stakeholder organizations. The standards are published in the *Palliative Care Certification Manual.*

Chapters address:

- Program management
- Provision of care, treatment, and services
- Information management
- Performance improvement

To be eligible for Advanced Certification for Palliative Care, a palliative care program must:

- Be provided within a TJC-accredited hospital. All types of hospitals are eligible, including children's hospitals and long-term acute care hospitals. A dedicated unit or dedicated beds are not required.
- Provide the full range of palliative care services to hospitalized patients 24 hours per day, seven days per week (24/7).
  - Programs must have team members available to answer phone calls nights and weekend and the ability to come to the hospital to see patients 24/7, when necessary, to meet patient and family needs.
  - Programs must be able to provide the same level of palliative care services during nights and weekends as during normal weekday hours.
  - Programs are not required to have palliative care team members physically present in the hospital 24/7.

Table 2.3 Consensus Recommendations: Operational Features for Hospital Palliative Care Programs

Domain	Recommendations		
	NQF*	Must Have	Should Have
1. Program administration To effectively integrate palliative care services into hospital culture and practice, so that the program's mission is aligned with that of the hospital, the program must have both visibility and voice within the hospital management structure. This can best be accomplished by (1) ensuring that a program has a designated program director, with dedicated funding for program director duties; and (2) a routine mechanism for program reporting and planning that is integrated into the hospital management committee structure.		Palliative care program staff integrated into the management structure of the hospital to ensure the program consideration of hospital mission and goals. Processes, outcomes, and strategic planning are developed in consideration of hospital mission and goals	Systems that integrate palliative care practices into the care of all seriously ill patients, not just those seen by the program
2. Types of services The three components of a fully integrated palliative care program are an inpatient consultation service, outpatient practice, and geographic inpatient unit. All three serve different, but complementary, functions to support patients and families through the illness experience. Because a consultation practice has the ability to serve patients throughout the entire hospital, this is typically recommended as the first point of program development.		A consultation service that is available to all hospital inpatients	Resources for outpatient palliative care services, especially in hospitals with more than 300 beds An inpatient palliative care geographic unit, especially in hospitals with more than 300 beds

(continued)

CHAPTER 2 **Hospital-Based Palliative Care**

Table 2.3 (Continued)

Domain	NQF*	Recommendations	
		Must Have	**Should Have**
3. Availability Patients, families, and hospital staff need palliative care services that are available for both routine and emergency services.	2	Monday to Friday inpatient consultation availability and 24/7 telephone support	24/7 inpatient consultation availability, especially in hospitals with more than 300 beds
4. Staffing The following disciplines are essential to provide palliative care services: physician, nursing, social work, and chaplaincy. In addition, mental health services must be available. Depending on the institution and staff, basic mental health screening services can be provided by an appropriately trained social worker, chaplain, or nurse with psychiatric training. Ideally, a psychologist or psychiatrist is also available for complex mental health needs. Social work, chaplaincy, and mental health services can be provided by dedicated palliative care full-time equivalent positions or by existing hospital staff, although their work in support of the palliative care program will still need to be accounted and paid for, and not just "added on" to their existing job responsibilities.	1, 5, 19, 20, 21, 22, 23	Specific funding for a designated palliative care physician All certified in hospice and palliative medicine (HPM) or committed to working toward board certification Specific funding for a designated palliative care nurse, with advance practice nursing preferred. All program nurses must be certified by the National Board for Certification of Hospice and Palliative Nursing (NBCHPN) or committed to working toward board certification. Appropriately trained staff to provide mental health services. Social worker and chaplain available to provide clinical care, as part of an interdisciplinary team Administrative support (secretary or administrative assistant position) in hospitals with either more than 150 beds or a consult service with volume of more than 15 consults per month	

5. Measurement	12, 13, 14, 15, 16	Operational metrics for all consultations. Customer, clinical and financial metrics that are tracked either continuously or intermittently
Providing evidence of the value of palliative care programs to patients, families, referring physicians, and hospital administrators is critical for program sustainability and growth. Key outcome measures can be divided into four domains (examples provided): • Operational metrics: (number of consults, referring physician, disposition) • Clinical metrics: (improvement in pain, dyspnea, distress) • Customer metrics: (patient, family, and referring physician satisfaction) • Financial metrics: (cost avoidance, billing revenue, length of stay)		
6. Quality improvement	12, 13, 14, 15, 16	Quality improvement activities, continuous or intermittent, for (a) pain, (b) nonpain symptoms, (c) psychosocial or spiritual distress, and (d) communication between healthcare providers and patients and/or surrogates
Palliative care programs must be held accountable to the same quality-improvement standards as other hospital clinical programs.		
7. Marketing		Marketing materials and strategies appropriate for hospital staff, patients, and families
As a new specialty, the palliative care program is responsible for making its presence and range of services known to the key stakeholders for quality care.		

(continued)

Table 2.3 (Continued)

Domain	NQF*	Recommendations	
		Must Have	**Should Have**
8. Education As a new specialty, the palliative care program is responsible for helping develop and coordinate educational opportunities and resources to improve the attitudes, knowledge, skills, and behavior of all health professionals.	3	Palliative care educational resources for hospital physicians, nurses, social workers, chaplains, health professional trainees, and any other staff members the program feels are essential to fulfill its mission and goals	
9. Bereavement services There are no currently accepted best practice features of bereavement services to recommend. Common elements present in many programs include telephone or letter follow-up, sympathy cards, registry of community resources for support groups and counseling services, and remembrance services. All programs are encouraged to develop a bereavement policy and make changes as needed through quality-improvement initiatives.	17, 30, 31	A bereavement policy and procedure that describes bereavement services provided to families of patients affected by the palliative care program	
10. Patient identification In most hospitals, palliative care consultations originate from a physician order. To facilitate referrals for "at-risk" patients, many hospitals have begun adopting screening.		A working relationship with the appropriate departments to adopt palliative care screening criteria for patients in the emergency department, general medical and surgical wards, and intensive care units	

11. Continuity of care Coordination of care as patients move from one care site to another is especially critical for patients with serious, life-limiting diseases and is a cornerstone of palliative care clinical work.	7, 8, 28	Policies and procedures that specify the manner in which transitions across care sites (e.g., hospital to home hospice) will be handled to ensure excellent communication between facilities A working relationship with one or more community hospice providers.
12. Staff wellness The psychological demands on palliative care staff are often overwhelming, placing practitioners at risk for burnout and a range of other mental health problems. Common examples of team wellness activities are team retreats, regularly scheduled patient debriefing exercises, relaxation and exercise training, and individual referral for staff counseling.	4	Policies and procedures that promote palliative care team wellness

The numbers in the NQF column represent the specific National Quality Forum Hospice and Palliative Medicine Preferred Practice. A National Framework and Preferred Practices for Palliative and Hospice Care Quality: A Consensus Report ©2006 National Quality Forum, www.qualityforum.org, Washington, DC.[23]

- Have served a minimum of 10 patients and have at least one active patient at the time of the initial TJC on-site review. Hospice patients are eligible for inclusion in the minimum patient count, only if they were receiving inpatient palliative care from the program before transitioning to hospice care. These patients may be selected for tracer activity during the on-site review, with the reviewer focusing on the episode of inpatient palliative care closest to the hospice transition.
- Use a standardized method of delivering clinical care, based on clinical practice guidelines and/or evidence-based practice
- Direct and coordinate the provision of palliative care, treatment, and services for the program patients (i.e., write orders, direct or coordinate activities of the patient care team, and influence composition of the patient care team)
- Follow an organized approach supported by an interdisciplinary team of health professionals
- Use performance measurement to improve its performance over time. Four months of performance measure data must be available at the time of the initial on-site certification review. At least two of the four measures must be clinical measures related to, or identified in, practice guidelines for the program. Measures selected by the program or service should be evidence-based, relevant, valid, and reliable. At this time, TJC is not defining the specific measures that are implemented; the emphasis is on the use of performance measures for improving palliative care services.
- Updates on TJC progress on standard development can be obtained from TJC website (http://www.jointcommission.org/certification/palliative_care.aspx) under "certification programs."

Professional Societies That Contribute to Palliative Care Development

Multiple professional societies have made contributions to the development of HBPC generalized or specialty population-specific palliative care standards, guidelines, or consensus statements by raising professional and public awareness of the unique issues of palliative care. A few selected organizations and their initiatives are described next.

National Hospice and Palliative Care Organization

The National Hospice and Palliative Care Organization (NHPCO) was founded in 1978 as the National Hospice Organization. The organization changed its name in February 2000 to include palliative care. Many hospice care programs added palliative care to their names to reflect the range of care and services they provide because hospice care and palliative care share the same core values and philosophies.

According to their website, the NHPCO is the largest, nonprofit membership organization representing hospice and palliative care programs and professionals in the United States. NHPCO is committed to improving EOL care and expanding access to hospice care, with the goal of profoundly enhancing quality of life for people dying in America and their loved ones. The NHPCO advocates for the terminally ill and their families. It also develops public and professional educational programs and materials to enhance understanding and availability of hospice and palliative care, convenes frequent meetings and symposia on emerging issues, provides technical informational resources to its membership, conducts research, monitors Congressional and regulatory activities, and works closely with other organizations that share an interest in EOL care.

Hospice and Palliative Nurses Association

Incorporated in 1987 as the Hospice Nurses Association, the Hospice and Palliative Nurses Association (HPNA) was created to establish a network and support for nurses in this specialty. In 1998, HPNA formally added palliative care to the organization to recognize the needs of nurses working in palliative care settings, separate from hospice. HPNA has become the nationally recognized organization providing resources and support for advanced practice nurses, registered nurses, licensed practical nurses, and nursing assistants, who care for people with life-limiting and terminal illness. As such, they have developed a number of position statements and standards to guide best practices that are available to members and non-members on a variety of topics.

Processes for Providing Hospital-Based Palliative Care

HBPC programs are increasing in number; however, many organizations are contemplating enhancing palliative resources or developing a program. Such an endeavor requires careful planning because these programs are not "one size fits all." Patience, persistence, and consensus-building are key elements to successful program development. As described earlier, CAPC has taken a leadership role in assisting organizations of all types to build a successful program that is suited to their unique patient population, resources, and organizational culture.

Particular to integrating palliative care principles into cancer centers through a multiyear grant, the City of Hope developed the Disseminating End of Life Education to Cancer Centers (DELETec).[25] In this multiyear project, they invited two-person teams to attend a three-day workshop conducted by nationally recognized, expert faculty to focus on best practices in palliative oncology care. The teams had additional follow-up support and assistance to help ensure successful program implementation. In all, 400 participants from 199 different cancer programs and institutions from 42 states attended one of their four programs.

A complete primer on developing an HBPC program is beyond the scope of this chapter; however, some of the most important care processes are described subsequently. Those wishing more complete information are referred to the excellent resources mentioned earlier in the chapter.

Program Development

Regardless of organizational type, the first step in developing an HBPC program is to perform a system assessment or "organizational scan" to identify existing organizational strengths, resources, potential partnerships, and collaborators. A task force or team of interested clinicians, administrators, and possibly consumers might be a good start. Examples of possible existing resources include clinicians from all disciplines with interest and training in palliative care, existing relationships with hospice, case management, discharge planners, and hospital chaplaincy programs. The needs assessment should determine the hospital focus on length of stay, ventilator days and pharmacy or ancillary costs per day, palliative care leadership based on personal experience or professional interest, preexisting pain programs, and trustee or philanthropic interest in and support for palliative care.

Second, after the system assessment is performed, identifying areas of need within the organization can highlight where palliative care programs can make the greatest contribution. Many institutions have easy access to data that can help to "build the case" for palliative care. Selling the idea of palliative care to an institution or gaining institutional support is more likely when benefits (e.g., economical, efficiency, improved clinical care) can be shown. Common areas of need that have shown improvement as a result of HBPC programs include pain and symptom management, patient and family satisfaction, nurse retention and satisfaction, bed and intensive care unit capacity, and length of stay. Other outcomes may include pharmacy costs, establishment and strengthening of hospice partnerships, and improvement of fragmented subspecialty care.

CAPC provides a Systems Assessment Tool and a Needs Assessment Checklist (http://www.capc.org/building-a-hospital-based-palliative-care-program/designing/system-assessment) to assist organizations with the complexities of the planning process.

Interdisciplinary Team Development

The holistic process of providing palliative care to patients and their families is rarely accomplished by one individual or discipline. The IDT is the foundation of the HBPC service and in many ways is unique in contrast to how medical care is traditionally provided. The core IDT typically consists of specially trained palliative care professionals, including physicians, nurses at all levels of training (registered nurses, nursing assistants, and advanced practice nurses [APNs]), social workers, pharmacists, spiritual care counselors, healing arts or complementary practitioners, hospice representatives, and volunteers.

Identifying which team members can best serve a patient's needs is a key part of the initial assessment. One clinician may be designated to receive initial consults and organize distribution of work for the day. A team may decide that all new consults are seen first by a medical provider: either the physician or APN. The physician also serves as the medical resource person for other team members and supervises physician learners. APNs may work independently or collaboratively with the attending physician to conduct initial consultations. If resources allow, this may be done together; however, workload and resources may dictate that new consults are divided among the medical providers.

In organizations that support learners, after a period of supervision and observation, it may be that the learner (e.g., fellow, resident, medical or nursing student) conducts an initial chart review and patient and/or family interview, and then presents the patient to the physician or APN—after which the pair will revisit the patient. At all times, the team should be aware of the patient's energy level and the learner's level of expertise in deciding if this format is appropriate. During the initial consult, the medical provider assesses psychological, social, and spiritual needs, and other team members are integrated into the plan of care.

A palliative care certified physician and/or APN may be responsible for the initial assessment and day-to-day medical care of most patients. However, depending on the patient's needs, another member of the team might take the lead in care. For example, if the patient's primary concern is physical, then a medical provider may direct the plan of care. If the patient's primary concern is existential in nature, the spiritual care provider may take the lead. Alternatively, if the patient's primary need is for family support, the social worker may be the most active care provider. Healing arts and complementary medicine practitioners and volunteers are also integral members of the IDT.

Healing arts and complementary medicine practitioners are providers from a variety of backgrounds who can provide massage, energy work, or instruction in guided imagery or meditation. Palliative care volunteers are specifically trained to see palliative care patients and are overseen by a volunteer coordinator. They provide presence, active listening, and company for patients and families. Although some tasks are seemingly small, such as reading, playing cards, or running small errands, these are often essential aspects of care from the patient and family perspective.

Pharmacists, healing arts and complementary therapy clinicians, hospice liaisons, and volunteers may or may not be part of the core team in some organizations. For example, even though medication needs may be complex, few teams have the ability to have a dedicated pharmacist who could round daily with the team. Hence, it may be more realistic to have a pharmacist present during regularly scheduled IDT meetings. Similarly, local hospice liaisons, healing arts and complementary therapy practitioners, and other providers may only be available to meet with a team weekly.

Nonclinical members of the team, including administrative, financial, or practice managers and secretarial support, are responsible for holding the IDT together by providing the supportive infrastructure within which the team can operate. These key team members may serve as representatives or liaisons on important institutional committees. Another important function of program administrators is the collection of data for clinical and fiscal evaluation for quality improvement, program justification to the institution, or research. The receptionist or secretarial support may be the first contact for patients and referring clinicians and can become the "face or voice of the program." Those selected for these positions should be skilled, patient, and caring individuals who can deal with the stress of people in crisis and with the urgency of consultations.

After an initial consultation, patients may continue to be seen in follow-up throughout their hospitalization. Some patients may have acute needs (e.g., uncontrolled pain) that may require them to be seen more than once daily. Other patients may be seen several times a week or weekly, or until the goal of the initial consultation is achieved. Some patients may be visited by the medical provider, the spiritual care provider, the healing arts provider, and a volunteer—all on the same day. In the case of Mr. X (see Box 2.1), visits from the palliative medicine provider and the spiritual care provider, among others, were frequent and provided the family with constant contact and opportunities to discuss concerns, feelings, or the simple comfort of another human presence.

Interdisciplinary Team Communication Support

Communication may be the most challenging and crucial aspect of providing palliative care. Intrateam communications that are regular and efficient will allow for seamless care to be delivered. Teams will likely explore a variety of mechanisms to achieve optimal communication about not only issues of patient care but also team function. The purpose of regular patient care–related team meetings is to allow all disciplines to contribute to the development and implementation of comprehensive care plans that reflect the values, preferences, goals, and needs of each individual patient.

Practicing as a true interdisciplinary team requires significant and ongoing intention and effort. Traditionally, the medical model has driven healthcare delivery and, to a large extent, still does. However, in a holistic care model of palliative care, the psychological, social, and spiritual care providers should have equal authority and input; for many clinicians, this represents a change in practice. Teams should be mindful of tendencies to become "efficient" that can sometimes lead to a focus only on the medical or physical aspects of care.

Minimally, a weekly face-to-face meeting, in which all IDT members gather, is considered an essential element of team function in order to provide high-quality, coordinated care. During the IDT meeting, active patients are presented, and all team members have an opportunity to contribute their expertise in the development of the plan of care. In some cases, weekly meetings may not be enough, and a team may choose to meet more frequently. These meetings are also a place to role-model, for the learners, healthy and respectful team interactions that recognize the value and expertise of each team member.

Performing the Palliative Care Consult

A palliative care consult can be initiated in a variety of different ways. Some services (or reimbursement mechanisms) require that a physician initiate the consult, rather than a nurse or other care provider. If someone other than the attending physician requests a consult on a hospitalized patient, it would still be important to include the attending (or primary care) physician in the consult. Ideally, a provider-to-provider conversation before consultation would be held to review and identify the priority issues. Most services choose to do this before seeing the patient.

When Is a Consult Made?

Consultations should be initiated any time a person with life-limiting illness has physical, psychological, social, or spiritual needs. Palliative care programs began for many reasons, but one of them was to meet the EOL care planning and symptomatic needs of patients who are not yet eligible for hospice, either because of life expectancy (greater than 6 months) or because they are receiving active disease-modifying treatment. Palliative care referrals do not hinge on the "less than 6 months" life expectancy, as is often the case for hospice referrals. Referring patients with life-limiting illness early is one of the benefits of having a palliative care service.

Some organizations have built-in consult triggers, protocols, or algorithms for specific life-limiting illnesses, in which consults are recommended at diagnosis. "Automatic referrals" would be generated for all patients who are newly diagnosed with certain types of life-limiting cancers (e.g., pancreatic, brain, stage IIIB and greater lung, or liver cancer). Noncancer patient populations that may be considered for automatic referrals are those with amyotrophic sclerosis, heart failure, or dialysis-dependent renal failure and those who, regardless of diagnosis, experience frequent hospitalizations. These patient populations are typically highly in need of palliative care services. Careful planning and close collaboration with colleagues is necessary to establish a process for automatic referrals that ensures that the patients most in need of palliative care services receive them "early and often." Some automatically scheduled palliative care consultations may occur in the outpatient setting or clinic, whereas some organizations have hospital "triggers" that may alert the primary team that a patient may benefit from these specialized services. Over time, in HBPC programs with high community visibility and/or marketing efforts, it may be common to have patients or family members self-refer.

What Is Included in the Initial Palliative Care Consultation?

The initial consult will lay the foundation for all further interactions with the patient and family (see Tables 2.2 and 2.3 and Figures 2.1 to 2.3). In addition to specialty expertise, the palliative care team may offer the unique resources

PALLIATIVE AND SUPPORTIVE MEDICINE CONSULT (PSMC)

(Worksheet only. Not part of permanent medical record.)

Medical Record Number: _____ **Age:** ___ **Reason for admission:** _____

To evaluate appropriateness of a PSMC, consider the following criteria:

SCORING

1. **Would you be surprised if this patient were alive in one year?**

Yes—score 3 points

No—score 0

TOTAL SECTION 1 (0 OR 3)

2. **Basic disease process**

Score 2 points each:

a. Cancer (metastatic/recurrent)

b. Advanced COPD (requires home oxygen)

c. Neurologic disease (difficulty swallowing or incontinent)

d. End-stage renal disease (considering stopping dialysis)

e. Advanced congestive heart failure (one-block DOE)

f. More than 3 hospitalizations or ED visits for incurable disease in past year

g. Other terminal or incurable disease causing significant symptoms

TOTAL SECTION 2

3. **Uncontrollable symptoms or clinical conditions**

Score 2 points each:	Score 1 point each:	Score 1 point each:
a. Pain	e. Anxiety	i. Prolonged vent support
b. Dyspnea	f. Depression	j. Other _____
c. Nausea	g. Weight loss	
d. Bowel obstruction	h. Constipation	
		TOTAL SECTION 3

4. **Anticipated functional status of patient at time of discharge**

Score as specified:

Using Eastern Cooperative Oncology Group (ECOG) Performance Status

Grade	Scale	Score
0–1	Fully active, able to carry on all predisease activities without restriction, or restricted in physically strenuous activity but ambulatory and able to carry out work of a light or sedentary nature	0
2	Ambulatory and capable of most self-care but unable to carry out any work activities; up and about more than 50% of waking hours	1
3–4	Capable of only limited self-care; confined to bed or chair more than 50% of waking hours or less	3

TOTAL SECTION 4 (0, 1, OR 3)

5. **Psychosocial issues (patient or family)**

Score 2 points each:

a. Need to discuss end of life issues

b. Need for evaluation for possible hospice referral

c. Artificial hydration or nutrition requested or considered

d. Unrealistic goals or expectations

TOTAL SECTION 5

TOTAL SCORE SECTIONS 1–5

SCORING GUIDELINES:

TOTAL SCORE ≤ 8   Problem-directed consult, if desired

TOTAL SCORE = 9–11   Consider PSMC

TOTAL SCORE ≥ 12   Strongly consider PSMC

Form completed by: _____ **Date:** _____

Figure 2.1 Palliative and supportive medicine consult (PSMC) tool.

PALLIATIVE AND SUPPORTIVE RAPID RESPONSE CONSULT (PMRRC)

(Worksheet only. Not part of permanent medical record.)

Medical Record Number: _____ **Age:** _____ **Reason for Admission:** _____

To evaluate appropriateness of a PMRRC, consider the following criteria:

1. Palliative medicine consult tool score > 9 (see page 1)
2. Patient referred from SNF for PEG tube placement with underlying significant dementia or progressive metastatic cancer

3. Patient older than 75 years with significant medical problems and:
    a. No advance directive and no surrogate decision-maker
    b. Advance directive that lists both *do* and *do not* selections
    c. Progressive single or multisystem disease with anticipated survival of one year or less and limited therapies available for the underlying disease
    d. Family or home caregivers with disparate goals for the patient
    e. Patient is full code and has multisystem organ failure, metastatic cancer, or a progressive terminal disease, despite treatment, or no treatment is planned for the underlying disease

4. Any suboptimally controlled acute post-trauma or postoperative pain problem
5. Any patient with cancer and pain
6. Patients or families who are requesting medical treatments for life prolongation or CPR that the primary service believes would be of little or no benefit to the patient
7. Assistance with medication logistics and discussion of possible hospice referral or comfort care plans for SNF

Figure 2.2 Palliative and supportive rapid response consult (PMRRC) tool.

Developed by Neil Ellison, MD, and Patricia Maani-Fogelman, DNP, Geisinger Health System.

of presence and time. Much has been written about the importance of setting during the initial consult.[6] Making sure there is adequate time to see the patient and family is crucial. If time restrictions are unavoidable, state these constraints at the outset of the consultation. Sitting down during the consultation and making sure everyone who is participating in the consult has a seat is important. Depending on the resources available and the composition of the team, an initial consult can occur almost anywhere. For inpatient consults, it is often in the patient's room; for outpatient consults, it may be in the clinic exam room. If resources permit, consults can also be done at patients' homes or in local care facilities. The main concern is an environment that allows for privacy and quiet—often difficult to find in most acute care hospitals.

Structure and Processes of Care

DARTMOUTH-HITCHCOCK MEDICAL CENTER

One Medical Center Drive

Lebanon, New Hampshire 03756

Physician/ARNP Order Sheet

Comfort Measures

Any order preceded by a check box must have the box checked to enable the order. All other orders will be automatically implemented.

☐ **DISCONTINUE ALL PREVIOUS ORDERS**

Activity: ☐ OOB as tolerated   ☐ OOB with assistance   ☐ Bed rest

Hunger: ☐ Diet as tolerated   ☐ NPO   ☐ Other _____

Thirst: ☐ PO Fluids as tolerated

IV fluids: ☐ No IVF   ☐ Yes _____

Dyspnea: ☐ O$_2$ prn for patient comfort   ☐ No oxygen   ☐ Fan at bedside

Elimination: ☐ Insert Foley catheter prn

Oral care: ☐ **per guideline (see reverse)**   ☐ **Other** _____

Skin care: ☐ **per guideline (see reverse)**   ☐ **Other** _____

Monitoring:

Vital signs: ☐ No   ☐ Yes—specify _____

Weight: ☐ No weights   ☐ Yes—specify _____

Labs: ☐ No lab draws   ☐ Yes—labs—specify _____

Consider Other Consults (if not already involved): ☐ Palliative care   ☐ Pastoral care

Medication for Symptom Management

Pain–scheduled (if PCA use special sheet):

Pain - breakthrough:

Dyspnea:

Anxiety/agitation:

Myoclonus:

Depression:

Sleep disturbance:

Pruritus:

Fever:

Nausea/vomiting:

Constipation:

Diarrhea:

Other orders:

Figure 2.3 Comfort measures orders sheet with guidelines for care as reference for staff education.
Source: Dartmouth-Hitchcock Medical Center, June 2004. Used with permission.

A generic equivalent may be administered when a drug has been prescribed by brand name unless the order states to the contrary.

_____   _____

Physician/ARNP   Signature Date/Time

_____   _____

Print Physician/ARNP Name   Pager or Phone

_____

Secretary Transcribing:

Original to the medical record P&T Committee: 7/15/2004 (P-225)

Yellow copy to Pharmacy Medical Records: 08/03/2004

See other side form #1826

Guidelines for Comfort Measures Orders

D/C ALL PREVIOUS ORDERS—Assess and reorder existing orders effective for comfort.

Activity: Goal is patient comfort. Activity level and hygiene routine should be based on patient's preference.

Hunger: Goal is to respond to patient's hunger, not to maintain a "normal nutritional intake."

Thirst: Goal is to respond to patient's thirst, which is best accomplished by oral fluids, sips, ice chips, and mouth care per patient desires, not IV hydration.

IV fluids: Goal is to avoid overhydration, which can lead to discomfort from edema, pulmonary and gastric secretions, and urinary incontinence. A small volume of IV fluid may assist with medication metabolism and delirium.

Dyspnea: Respond to the patient's perception of breathlessness rather than "numerical abnormalities"—i.e., oxygen saturation via pulse oximetry. Interventions include medications (e.g., opioids, antianxiety agents, steroids), scopolamine patch, and minimizing IV fluids to decrease secretions; oxygen therapy per nasal cannula prn for patient comfort—avoid facemask.

Fans at bedside: Fans are available for patient comfort and are often more effective for perception of breathlessness than other interventions.

Elimination: Focus on managing distress from bowel or bladder incontinence. Insert Foley catheter prn, per patient comfort and desire.

Oral care: Studies show dry mouth is the most common and distressing symptom in conscious patients at end of life.

Provide ice chips and sips of fluid prn; humidify oxygen to minimize oral/nasal drying.

Provide mouth care every 2 hours and prn—sponge oral mucosa and apply lubricant to lips and oral mucosa.

Skin care: Air mattress, pressure sore prevention measures per DHMC skin care guidelines. Incontinent care every 2 hours and prn.

Monitoring: Focus monitoring on the patient's symptoms (e.g., pain) and responses to comfort measures.

Psychosocial consults: Goal is to provide resources and support through the dying process.

Medication for symptom management (scheduled and PRN):

Pain management, scheduled and breakthrough: consider PCA/IV/SQ/rectal analgesics.

Dyspnea management: consider opioids, scopolamine patch, atropine for secretions.

Anxiety/agitation management: consider combination of lorazepam (Ativan) and haloperidol (Haldol).

Figure 2.3 continued

Myoclonus: consider benzodiazepines and/or opioid rotation for myoclonus.

Depression management: evaluate for antidepressants or methylphenidate.

Sleep disturbance management: consider diphenhydramine (Benadryl).

Pruritus management: consider diphenhydramine (Benadryl) PO/IV.

Fever management: consider acetaminophen (Tylenol) PO/rectal.

Nausea/vomiting management: consider prochlorperazine (Compazine), metoclopramide; 5-HT3 antagonist PO/IV.

Constipation management: consider narcotic bowel orders.

Diarrhea management: consider diphenoxylate/atropine (Lomotil) or loperamide (Imodium).

Figure 2.3 continued

References

1. Teno JM, Gozalo PL, Bynum JW, et al. Change in end of life care for Medicare beneficiaries: site of death, place of care, and healthcare transitions in 2000, 2005, and 2009. *JAMA*. 2013;309(5):470–477.

2. Goodman DC, Esty AR, Fisher ES, Chang C-H. Trends and variation in end of life care for Medicare beneficiaries with severe chronic illness: a report of the Dartmouth Atlas Project. http://www.dartmouthatlas.org/downloads/reports/EOL_Trend_Report_0411.pdf. Accessed October 2, 2014.

3. Bercovitz A, Decker FH, Jones A, Remsburg RE. End of life care in nursing homes: 2004 National Nursing Home Survey. *Natl Health Stat Rep*. 2008;9:1–24.

4. Smith AK, McCarthy E, Weber E, et al. Half of older Americans seen in emergency department in last month of life: most admitted to hospital, and many die there. *Health Aff*. 2012;31:1277–1285.

5. Bailey FA, Williams BR, Goode PS, et al. Opioid pain medication orders and administration in the last days of life. *J Pain Symptom Manage*. 2012;44(5):681–691.

6. Berwick DM. The science of improvement. *JAMA*. 2008;299(10): 1182–1184.

7. Center to Advance Palliative Care. 2011 Public opinion research on palliative care: a report based on research by public opinion strategies. http://www.capc.org/tools-for-palliative-care-programs/marketing/public-opinion-research/2011-public-opinion-research-on-palliative-care.pdf. Accessed October 2, 2014.

8. Weissman DE, Meier DE. Center to advance palliative care inpatient unit operational metrics: consensus recommendations. *J Palliat Med*. 2009;12(1):21–25.

9. World Health Organization. *Cancer Pain Relief and Palliative Care*. Geneva: World Health Organization; 1990.

10. Ajemian I, Mount B. *The Royal Victoria Hospital Manual on Palliative/Hospice Care: A Resource Book*. Montreal: Palliative Care Service: Royal Victoria Hospital; 1980.

11. Temel JS, Greer JA, Muzikansky A, et al. Early palliative care for patients with metastatic non–small-cell lung cancer. *N Engl J Med*. 2010;363:733–742.

12. Center to Advance Palliative Care, National Palliative Care Research Center. *America's Care of Serious Illness: A State-by-State Report Card on Access to Palliative Care in Our Nation's Hospitals*. New York: Center to Advance Palliative Care; 2008:34.

13. Goldsmith B, Dietrich J, Qingling D, Morrison RS. Variability in access to hospital palliative care in the United States. *J Palliat Med*. 2008;11:1094–1102.

14. Center to Advance Palliative Care, National Palliative Care Research Center. *Building a Hospital Based Palliative Care Program*. http://www.capc.org/building-a-hospital-based-palliative-care-program. Accessed October 2, 2014.

15. O'Mahoney S, Blank AE, Zallman L, Selwyn P. The benefits of a hospital-based inpatient palliative care consultation service: preliminary outcome data. *J Palliat Med*. 2008;8:1033–1039.

16. Teno JM. Palliative care teams: self-reflection—past, present, and future. *J Pain Symptom Manage*. 2002;23:94–95.

17. Higginson I, Finlay I, Goodwin D, et al. Do hospital-based palliative teams improve care for patients or families at the end of life? *J Pain Symptom Manage*. 2001;23:96–106.

18. Dunlop RJ, Hockley JM. *Terminal Care Support Teams*. New York: Oxford University Press; 1990.

19. Claessen SJ, Francke AL, Belarbi HE, et al. A new set of quality indicators for palliative care: process and results of the development trajectory. *J Pain Symptom Manage*. 2011;42:169–182.

20. Zimmermann C, Riechelmann R, Krzyzanowska M, et al. Effectiveness of specialized palliative care: a systematic review. *JAMA*. 2008;299:1698–1709.

21. Smith TJ, Coyne P, Cassel B, et al. A high-volume specialist palliative care unit and team may reduce in-hospital end of life care costs. *J Palliat Med*. 2003;6:699–705.

22. Rabow M, Dibble S, Pantilat S, McPhee S. The comprehensive care team: a controlled trial of outpatient palliative medicine consultation. *Arch Intern Med*. 2004;164:83–91.

23. National Quality Forum. *A National Framework and Preferred Practices for Palliative and Hospice Care Quality: A Consensus Report*. Washington, DC: National Quality Forum; 2006.

24. The Joint Commission. *Certification for Palliative Care Programs*. 2013. http://www.jointcommission.org/certification/palliative_care.aspx. Accessed October 2, 2014.

25. Grant M, Hanson J, Mullan P, et al. Disseminating end of life education to cancer centers: overview of program and of evaluation. *J Cancer Educ*. 2007;22:140–148.

Chapter 3

Home Care and Hospice Care

Marilyn Bookbinder and Romina Arceo

Palliative home care can be used for chronically ill patients to improve their quality of life. Often, home care interventions can be provided on a short-term basis when clients experience a crisis that requires focused interventions.

Nurses are the leaders and essential members of the home care team. Advanced practice nurses (APNs) can have an impact on the cost, access to, and quality of care provided to chronically ill patients.

Patients with complex problems need family caregivers who are taught to provide care in the home. Caregiving can be extremely stressful for family members and may adversely affect the health of the caregiver. Home care providers should assist family caregivers to maintain their health.

Palliative home care should be provided by a team of providers, including physicians, mental health workers, therapists, nurses, and paraprofessionals.

Originally, palliative care in home care nursing was associated with patients who were clearly near the end of life. The contemporary philosophy of palliative care had its beginnings in England in 1967, when Dame Cicely Saunders founded St. Christopher's Hospice. Home and respite care continue to be a major component of that program. Palliative care, by definition, focuses on the multidimensional aspects of patients and families, including physical, psychological, social, spiritual, and interpersonal components of care. These components of care need to be instituted throughout all phases of the chronic illness trajectory and not only at the point when patients qualify for hospice services. Palliative care also needs to be given across a variety of settings and not be limited to inpatient units.

The primary purpose of palliative care is to enhance the quality and meaning of life and death for both patients and loved ones. To-date, health professionals have not used the potential of palliative care to maximize the quality of life of patients in their homes. In this chapter, we discuss home care as an environment that provides unique opportunities to promote palliative care for patients and families throughout their illness.

Definition of Home Care Nursing

Home care, home healthcare, and home care nursing can be confusing terms to both providers and consumers because they are often used interchangeably. Numerous definitions of home care have been provided by the many professional and trade associations that address home care issues (e.g., National Association for Home Care, Consumer's Union, American Hospital Association, American Medical Association, Center for Medicare and Medicaid Services). Common to all the definitions is the recognition that home care is care of the sick and well in the home by professionals and paraprofessionals, with the goal to improve health, enhance comfort, and improve the quality of life of clients. Home care nursing is defined here as ". . . the provision of nursing care to acutely ill, chronically ill, terminally ill, and well patients of all ages in their residences. Home care nursing focuses on health promotion and care of the sick while integrating environmental, psychosocial, economic, cultural, and personal health factors affecting an individual's and family's health status."[1]

Home Care Use in the United States

Home care is a diverse industry that provides a broad scope of care to patients of all ages. In 2010, it was estimated that approximately 12 million people received home care services for acute illness, long-term health conditions, permanent disability, and terminal illness.[2] The demographic picture of home healthcare recipients shows a predominately female (63.8%) and white (90.3%) population. The majority (86.1%) of home care patients are age 65 years and older, although home care is provided to patients of all ages, from birth to death. By 2050, it is estimated that 27 million people will need long-term care, the majority of which will be provided in the home. The number of elderly people receiving home care is expected to increase in the coming years because of the aging of the American population and the desire of individuals to age in place.[3]

Although home care is provided to a large number of people, it still represents a very small percentage of national healthcare expenditures. Home care represented only 3% of the total national health expenditure in 2009, whereas hospital care consumed 37% and physician services 26%,[2] demonstrating the cost-efficient nature of home care practice. The majority of patients (67.5%) who received home care were discharged primarily to urban home care agencies.[3] As the reimbursement for home care visits has decreased (Table 3.1) and the cost of home visiting in rural areas has increased because of increased travel time, many rural home care agencies have been forced to close, limiting access to home care for the population in the region. The federal government has been inconsistent in its payment of additional dollars to home care agencies that provide care in rural settings.

The most common primary diagnosis for home care patients is diseases of the circulatory system, including heart disease. Other common primary

Table 3.1 Criteria for Home Care Reimbursement Under Medicare

Criterion	Description
Homebound	A patient is considered homebound if absences from the home are rare, short of duration, and attributable to the need to receive medical treatments.
Completed plan of care	A plan of care for home care services must be completed in Centers for Medicare and Medicaid services (CMS) forms 485 and 487. The plan of care must be signed by a physician.*
Skilled service	Medicare defines skilled service as one provided by a registered nurse, physical therapist, or speech therapist. Skilled nursing services include skilled observation and assessment, teaching, direct care and management, and evaluation of the plan of care.
Intermittent and part-time	Part-time means that skilled care and home health aide services combined may not exceed 8 hours per day or 28 hours per week. Intermittent means that skilled care is provided or needed on fewer than 7 days per week or less than 8 hours of each day for periods of 21 days or less, with extensions for exceptional circumstances.
Reasonable and necessary	The services provided must be reasonable for the patient given the diagnosis and necessary to assist the patient to achieve the expected outcomes.

diagnoses of patients receiving home care are diseases of the musculoskeletal system and connective tissue; diabetes mellitus; diseases of the respiratory system; endocrine, nutritional, and metabolic diseases; and immunity disorders.[2] Home care patients have an average of 4.2 diagnoses at the time of admission to an agency. A primary diagnosis of malignant neoplasm represents only 3.9% of home healthcare patients,[3] whereas it accounts for 47% of all patients in hospice. Clearly, nonhospice home care has not been used adequately as an integral part of care for cancer patients and families as they have endured the physical and emotional demands of complex cancer treatments and move across the acute, chronic, and terminal phases of their disease. This is an ideal context in which the need for palliative care should drive an increased use of home care services.

Recommendations for Facilitating the Use of Home Care Nursing in Palliative Care

Home care nursing is an ideal mechanism to deliver effective palliative care; however, for a number of reasons, it has been underused. Patients who need palliative care have complex and often challenging physical and psychological problems. Palliative care for specific types of diseases requires knowledgeable and competent clinicians. It is common for professional staff nurses in home care agencies to lack the knowledge and expertise to manage patients' symptoms and to teach caregivers the skills they need to manage the day-to-day problems they encounter in caregiving. And yet repeatedly, home care nurses are placed in the position of being responsible for patients who have palliative care needs. One potential solution is to teach the staff to use evidence-based research to remain current in the advances in palliative care. The rationale for promoting evidence-based palliative care is straightforward, but there are major challenges to achieving the goal of translating palliative care research into everyday clinical practice. Maybe the most difficult challenge is persuading the staff to change how they deliver care.[4] Schumacher and colleagues used standard pain management strategies to teach the staff to change their practice in the home.[5] Another successful strategy has been the use of medication kits, containing prescription medications to treat pain and dyspnea, for use with dying patients as they approach death.[6] In addition, for palliative care to be successful in the home, physicians and other experts must work collaboratively with nurses and be available to solve problems as they arise. It is often easier for physicians to admit patients to the hospital than to work with home care nurses to keep patients at home.

The state of the science in home care was reviewed for this chapter. Results from these studies have not been systematically incorporated into clinical practice where services are reimbursed. However, we identified critical factors in these studies that, if adopted, could become the basis of successful home care palliative nursing. These include the following:

1. Staff nurses who are responsible for direct patient care in the home must have contact with experts who have specialized knowledge and skills related to the disease-specific needs of patients. Experts can include any member of a palliative care program, but usually include an APN or palliative care physician. An APN is defined here as a professional nurse, including clinical nurse specialists and nurse practitioners, who has graduated from a master's program in a specialty field such as an oncology advanced practice program. To assist the staff nurse in dealing with the complexity of palliative care, either a palliative care physician or an APN should serve as a supervisor/consultant to the team and be directly involved in clinical decisions. There may be fewer than needed opportunities for APNs working directly in home care agencies because of the perception that they are too costly to employ. As agencies move to prospective payment and greater efficiency, the role of the APN may factor more prominently in home care agencies. APNs may also work independently and provide care to a group of patients, such as case managers from an ambulatory clinic. As a result of the Balanced Budget Act of 1997 (PL 105–55), APNs—specifically clinical nurse specialists and nurse practitioners—practicing in any setting can be directly reimbursed at 85% of the physician fee schedule for services provided to Medicare beneficiaries. In home care, this change has the potential to facilitate access to care for patients who do not have access to a home care agency or other primary care provider, specifically those in rural and underserved areas.

2. Because of the barriers to entering hospice care, home care nurses must become knowledgeable and highly skilled in providing palliative care to patients. This will require not only the development of skills in a new area of clinical expertise but also a paradigm shift in the way home care nurses view the episode of care for patients in the home. Home care has traditionally been viewed as a component of the long-term care delivery system. Although the number of home visits per episode of illness has decreased significantly, home visits tend to be spread out over a greater period of time, usually a 60-day certification period. For patients requiring palliation, home care may need to be very intensive over a relatively short period of time (2 to 4 weeks). In this model, the home care nurse can assist the patient and family in methods of managing symptoms and coping with the caregiving role. In the long term, as the patient's disease progresses, the patient and caregivers will need "booster" visits, but the majority of visits and care may be given in short periods of time, when the patient and caregivers are most in need. Telephone visits to provide care have been shown to be an effective strategy for chronic illnesses in which the needs are for support and education. Home care can also be used for short durations in crisis situations. By providing intensive home care for short durations, patients can be helped to address current issues in the most effective way. These short but intensive interventions can improve quality of life and may also affect survival outcomes for some patients. Although home health agencies are usually paid on the basis of a 60-day episode of care, the prospective payment system (PPS) has a low-utilization payment for beneficiaries whose episode of care consists of four or fewer visits.[7]

3. Patients are usually hospitalized when symptoms get out of control and their disease is unstable. When patients are hospitalized, comprehensive discharge care coordination and follow-up by nurses skilled in palliative care is needed to ensure that the plan is implemented, evaluated, and modified, as needed. Patients with complex problems, including distressing symptoms, need assistance to make a smooth transition from the hospital to their home, and caregivers need access to information, skills training, and resources to help with providing essential assistance. A referral to a home care agency may also be necessary for successful outcomes. The complexity of symptom management following hospitalization may require the advanced skills of an APN or other expert in palliative care to provide consultation to the home care nurse or to implement a plan of care with a patient and family. Access to these nurses may be based in a variety of settings, such as hospital-based clinics, private offices, and home care agencies. The multidisciplinary care provided by nurses, physicians, paraprofessionals, social workers, chaplains, and pharmacists is essential to the development of positive outcomes. As members of the multidisciplinary team, physicians must work in collaboration with other professionals across settings to provide comprehensive care to patients and families. Collaboratively, the team determines the amount of care needed, the most

appropriate setting for care, and the type of interventions required to improve the patient's quality of life.

4. Patients who have complex problems and receive home care nursing need family caregivers who are willing and able to learn the skills to provide care. Standardized educational programs to teach family caregivers skills to provide care are needed and should be a part of routine home nursing care. Examples of successful evidence-based programs have been cited in this chapter and can serve as an excellent beginning for nurses in home care facilities to develop a program. In the event these caregivers are ill themselves, additional or complementary services need to be provided to help with the patients' care. Nurses providing home care for ill patients should conduct ongoing assessments of family caregivers, including willingness and skills to provide care, their health, and demands made on them.

5. The use of innovative models must be considered as a strategy for providing care to patients and families. Telephone visits have been shown to be an effective strategy to help families cope with the caregiver role. Traditionally, specific criteria have been used to define the requirements for home care services. These criteria need to be reexamined in light of our increased understanding of disease patterns, treatment effects, and patient responses to illness. In the future, we need to consider alternative ways of delivering services to patients and family caregivers. Telephone contacts have been shown to be an effective strategy to help families cope with the caregiver role. Under prospective payment for home care, home care providers are no longer constrained by the per-visit method of reimbursement, and telephone visits can be integrated into the plan of care. The use of alternative and complementary therapy, nutritional counseling, or mental health therapies has been made financially reasonable as a result of the move to prospective payment. Telehealth programs have also been used effectively with patient populations at home. Other technology interventions could include the use of the Internet or e-mail.[8,9] As the technology becomes less expensive, increased opportunity to implement these strategies will be available.

A growing number of cancer patients are being discharged from the hospital after surgery or other cancer treatments to be cared for at home by family caregivers who have chronic illnesses themselves, as described by the following case study (Box 3.1). In this case study, we illustrate how patients can be admitted and discharged several times to home care, throughout their illness trajectory. It is well established that patients can obtain the greatest benefit from palliative care, if it is instituted early as part of their home care.

Box 3.1 Case Study: Mr. D

Trajectory Point 1 (Diagnostic and Hospital Phase)

Mr. D is a 61-year-old executive who has worked his entire life to provide for his wife and three grown children. Overall, he had been in good health, monitoring his cholesterol and blood pressure since both his parents died of cardiac disease. During the past decade, he gradually gained weight because of his sedentary lifestyle, extended working hours, and increased dependency of his wife, who was diagnosed with multiple sclerosis eight years ago.

About a month ago, Mr. D began having indigestion and heart burn. After ruling out cardiac problems, his primary care physician ordered antireflux medications. Subsequently, he complained of persistent pain, bloating, and difficulty getting his breath. A referral to the gastroenterologist revealed he had a large mass at the base of the esophagus. Because of the size of the tumor, it was recommended that Mr. D undergo radiation therapy to reduce the tumor before surgery. After completing six weeks of radiation treatment, Mr. D underwent removal of the distal end of his esophagus. Preoperatively, Mr. D experienced acute anxiety over his fear of being unable to care for his wife. His eldest daughter had come to care for her mother during his hospitalization, but she needed to leave to care for her own family and to return to work. Mr. D's postoperative recovery proceeded smoothly; he resumed a regular diet and was able to ambulate without assistance, and his pain was well controlled. During his hospital stay, he and his family met with a social worker to identify needs after discharge. Because of his improving health, he reported less anxiety about his wife but identified a new concern related to his diagnosis of advanced cancer and requirement for additional cancer treatment. His return to nearly normal physical functioning and improved control of symptoms, however, resulted in his discharge after four days with routine postoperative instructions and no referral for home care services. He woke during his first night at home with severe pain and difficulty breathing. His wife called 911, and he was subsequently rehospitalized and diagnosed with a pulmonary embolus.

During his second hospitalization, Mr. D was treated for his pulmonary embolus. He also reported increased pain related to swallowing, prompting a consult to the palliative care service. During this time, the palliative care advance practice nurse (APN) recommended changes to his pain medications. He was also taught to administer his anticoagulation medication subcutaneously and was assisted by a nurse discharge coordinator to arrange home nursing services; he was considered homebound and in need of skilled nursing services. The goals of this skilled care were to ensure his safe administration of subcutaneous anticoagulation medication, help stabilize his blood coagulation, monitor signs and symptoms related to his potential for a recurrent embolus, and provide ongoing monitoring of his postoperative recovery, particularly his pain. As part of her skilled observation and assessment, the home care nurse identified

(continued)

Box 3.1 (Continued)

a potentially unstable situation due to Mr. D's role as primary caregiver for his wife and counseled the couple to consider arranging for home-maker services for Mrs. D., if Mr. D's condition was to worsen temporarily because of his ongoing cancer treatment with chemotherapy.

Trajectory Point 2 (Treatment)

Within four weeks after the second hospitalization, Mr. D's need for skilled nursing services lessened: he was able to return to work, his incision had healed, his stamina had improved, he was transitioned from subcutaneous anticoagulation medication to oral therapy, and his blood coagulation studies were considered within a therapeutic range. His throat pain had improved, and he was able to reduce his reliance on the analgesics. Home care services were discontinued, even though Mr. D's medical oncologist recommended he have a six-month course of chemotherapy to reduce his chance of recurrence. Mr. D agreed and attempted to work full-time during his treatment and care full-time for his ailing wife. Eventually, his cumulative chemotherapy treatments resulted in increasing fatigue, issues with neutropenia, and persistent and progressive neuropathic symptoms. He reported to his medical oncologist how his symptoms had resulted in a reduced work schedule because he was unable to care for both his wife and do his job. He also reported that his anxiety had returned and he was having trouble sleeping. His medical oncologist contacted the palliative care team again. Mr. D met with a palliative care APN who recommended changes to his medications and self-management strategies to improve control of his physical and emotional symptoms. Also, she collaborated with the institution-based oncology nurse case manager to implement home health aide and home-maker services for his wife.

Trajectory Point 3 (Survivorship)

Once Mr. D's symptoms lessened, he gradually returned to work full-time and to his caregiving duties. He was discharged from the palliative care service. Mr. D remained asymptomatic and without any evidence of disease for 18 months.

Trajectory Point 4 (Initial Recurrence)

Over time, Mr. D found he was losing weight, had a poor appetite, and had become increasingly tired. His subsequent magnetic resonance image demonstrated that the mass had returned and had spread to his liver. Mr. D and his family agreed to more chemotherapy to treat the symptoms associated with the return and spread of his cancer. Even with his chemotherapy, his symptoms were not adequately controlled. He continued to experience more intense weakness and loss of appetite. He developed abdominal ascites, difficulty swallowing, difficulty breathing, and generalized pain. His anxiety had also returned because of his decline

(continued)

Box 3.1 (Continued)

in physical health. Despite his increasing physical dependency, Mr. D wanted to remain at home. The palliative care APN instituted palliative care services in the home, consisting of skilled nursing visits, home health aide support, and counseling by a palliative care social worker and pastoral staff. Mr. D's plan of care included pain management, nutritional and bowel management, support with activities of daily living, and counseling as it pertained to his job, finances, health insurance coverage issues, advance directives, and role as primary caregiver. Mr. D's social worker and the pastoral staff also spent time with him and his family preparing them for the inevitable outcome.

Trajectory Point 5 (End of Life)

Mr. D became increasingly sedentary and symptomatic, causing his medical oncologist and his palliative care APN to initiate a discussion about stopping chemotherapy treatments. Mr. D and his family agreed. This change in treatment enabled Mr. D to be eligible for hospice-level benefits and hospice-level services at home. Fortunately, the home care agency providing services to Mr. D was certified as a hospice care agency, thereby allowing Mr. D and his family to keep the same home care providers. Within days, Mr. D's home care nurses assessed his progression toward dying and supported his decline accordingly. Two weeks after his death, Mr. D's palliative care APN met with the family to review the care that Mr. D had received. The nurse reinforced what a good job the family did with helping to keep Mr. D at home throughout his illness. Up to six months after his death, the palliative care APN kept in touch with the family to assist with their bereavement.

References

1. American Nurses Association. *Home Health Nursing: Scope and Standards of Practice.* Silver Springs, MD: American Nurses Association; 2008.

2. National Association for Home Care. *Basic Statistics About Home Care.* Updated 2010. http://www.nahc.org/assets/1/7/10HC_Stats.pdf. Accessed October 27, 2014.

3. U.S. Department of Health and Human Services. *Home Health Care and Discharged Hospice Care Patients: United States, 2000–2007.* National Health Statistics Reports Number 38, Washington, DC: 2011.

4. Jacobosen P. Promoting evidence-based psychosocial care for cancer patients. *Psycho-Oncology.* 2009;18:6–13.

5. Schumacher KL, Koresawa S, West C, et al. Putting cancer pain management regimens into practice at home. *J Pain Symptom Manage.* 2002;23:369–382.

6. Bishop M, Stephens L, Goodrich M, Byock I. Medication kits for managing symptomatic emergencies in the home: a survey of common hospice practice. *J Palliat Med.* 2009;12:37–43.

7. Center for Medicare and Medicaid Services. *Home Health PPS*. http://www.cms.gov/Medicare/Medicare-Fee-for-Service-Payment/HomeHealthPPS/index.html. Accessed October 2, 2014.

8. Bowles K, Baigh A. Applying research evidence to optimize telehomecare. *J Cardiovasc Nurs*. 2007;22(1):5–15.

9. Kinsella, A, Doughty, K. Home telehospice: new tools for end of life care services. *J Assist Technol*. 2009,2:47–50.

Chapter 4

The Intensive Care Unit

Jennifer McAdam and Kathleen Puntillo

An intensive care unit (ICU) is, by tradition, the setting in which the most aggressive care is rendered to hospitalized patients. Patients are admitted to an ICU so that health professionals can perform minute-to-minute titration of care. The primary goals of this aggressive care are patient resuscitation, stabilization, and recovery from the acute phase of an illness or injury. However, many patients die in ICUs. It is estimated that greater than 500,000 people die after admission to ICUs in the United States each year.[1] Stated otherwise, almost one in five Americans receives ICU services before death. Researchers assessing mortality rates in seven states found that 47% of all hospital deaths involved intensive care services.[2] Investigators comparing Medicare beneficiaries' places of care and sites of death from 2000 to 2009 reported a significant increase in ICU use during the last 30 days of life, with 29% of the decedents experiencing ICU care in the last month of life.[3] In addition, 24% of patients with poor-prognosis cancers were admitted to the ICU within 30 days of death.[4] Therefore, it is clear that management of the process of dying is common in ICUs.

In the high-technology environment of an ICU, it may be difficult for health professionals and families of dying patients to acknowledge that there are limits to the effectiveness of medical care. However, it is important to focus on providing the type of care that is appropriate for the individual patient and the patient's family, be it aggressive life-saving care, palliative care that includes symptom management, good communication, and interdisciplinary collaboration, or palliative end of life care. This chapter discusses the provision of palliative care in ICUs, with an emphasis on end of life care. Specifically, challenges and barriers to providing such care in ICUs are described, and recommendations are offered for the provision of symptom assessment and management. Current issues related to holding family meetings, establishing patient goals of care, surrogate decision-making, and withholding and withdrawing life-sustaining therapies are covered. Recommendations are offered for attending to the needs of families as well as healthcare providers who care for ICU patients at the end of life. Finally, an international agenda for improving end of life care in ICUs is presented.

Limitations of End of Life Care in Intensive Care Units

Although many deaths occur in ICUs, an ICU is rarely the place that one would choose to die. Health professionals in ICUs, frequently uncertain about whether a patient will live or die, are caught between the opposing goals of preserving life and preparing the patient and family for death. It is important for professionals to realize that a patient's death is not necessarily an indication of ineffective care. Yet, there remain serious limitations to the care provided to seriously ill and dying patients and their families. Communication between physicians, patients, and family members may be poor[5]; patients and family members may be overly optimistic about the outcomes of cardiopulmonary resuscitation (CPR) and have unrealistic expectations of ICU technologic treatments; end of life decision-making can be challenging and present conflicts; and many hospitalized patients die in moderate to severe pain and with other troubling symptoms.[6]

In a landmark study, more than 5,000 seriously ill hospitalized patients or their family members were asked questions about the patients' pain (SUPPORT).[7] Almost one half of these patients had pain during the previous 3 days, and almost 15% had pain that was moderately or extremely severe and occurred at least half of the time. Of those with pain, 15% were dissatisfied with its control. In a more recent study measuring the symptom experiences of 171 ICU patients at high risk for dying, symptom prevalence ranged from 27% (confused) to 75% (tired), and many symptoms were reported as intense (thirst) and distressful (shortness of breath, scared, confused, and pain).[6] In a retrospective chart review of 88 ICU patients with advanced cancer referred for palliative care consultation, a significant proportion reported symptoms such as pain (84%), dyspnea (82%), fatigue (95%), constipation (60%), anxiety (65%), and depression (45%).[8] These findings stress the importance of attending to the assessment and management of pain and other symptoms in all ICU patients.

Planning Palliative Care for Intensive Care Unit Patients

Providing comfort to patients should accompany all ICU care, even during aggressive attempts to prolong life. However, if a patient is not expected to survive, the focus shifts to an emphasis on palliative care. It is often extremely difficult in an ICU to determine the appropriate time for a change of focus in care. A transition period occurs during which the health professionals, the patient's family, and sometimes the patient recognize the appropriateness of withdrawing and/or withholding life-sustaining treatments and begin to make preparations for death. The transition period (i.e., the time from decision to death) may be a matter of minutes or hours, as in the case of a patient who has sustained massive motor vehicle collision injuries, or it may be a matter of weeks, as in the case of a patient who has undergone bone marrow transplantation and has multiple negative sequelae while in the ICU. Clearly, this time difference must be recognized as a factor that can influence the experience of a patient's family members. When patients rapidly approach death, their family members may not have time to overcome the shock of the trauma and adjust to the possibility of death. On the other hand, when death is prolonged, family frustration and fatigue may be part of their experience. Health professionals who are sensitive to these different experiences can individualize their approaches and interventions for family members.

The death trajectory in the ICU usually follows one of these patterns: a patient in good health who suffers a catastrophic event such as an intracranial bleed; a patient with several comorbidities who presents with a new acute problem; a patient with an exacerbation of a chronic condition; or an elderly patient progressively declining with a life-threatening illness. However, the transition from aggressive care to death preparation has not been well operationalized. The transition period is clearly uncomfortable for many healthcare professionals because clinically useful prediction models, recognizing which patients have the highest risk for death in the ICU, remain elusive. Scenarios concerning end of life decision-making in the absence of patient or family input are especially challenging. Therefore, it is important for ICU professionals to hold patient and family meetings early in the ICU stay in order to address goals of care. The following steps may be useful when caring for patients at risk for not surviving their ICU course:

- Ascertain whether the patient has developed an advance directive, whether a family member has durable power of attorney, and whether the patient has communicated a preference about CPR. In a retrospective review of 347 patients who died in the ICU, only 22% of the patients' preferences regarding life support were documented, and in 36% of the cases, it was not reported whether a patient's representative existed or was involved with decision-making.[9]

- Hold a patient and family meeting early in the ICU stay with the goal being within the first five days.[10] Identify and communicate the goals of care for the patient and discuss and update them daily.

- Outline the steps that need to be taken to accomplish the goals of care and evaluate their effectiveness. Technology should not drive the goals of care. Instead, technology should be used, when necessary, to accomplish the goals, and its use should be minimized when the primary goal is achievement of a peaceful death. Use a multidisciplinary team approach to decision-making regarding transition to end of life care. All team members, including the patient's family, should reach a consensus—sometimes through negotiation—that the withdrawal of life support and a peaceful death are the appropriate patient outcomes.[11]

- In a situation in which the patient lacks decision-making capacity and surrogate representation, it is recommended that a court appoint a guardian on behalf of the patient or that safeguards be put in place to protect the patient's interests, such as a mandatory ethics committee review. It is generally not recommended that the physician make the decision in isolation.[11]

- Develop and communicate the palliative care plan to professionals and family and identify the best persons for implementing the various actions in the plan. Developing a plan of care may include enlisting the assistance of in-hospital palliative care staff and/or hospice services. The major goals in any palliative care plan are to provide optimal symptom management, provide psychosocial and spiritual support, provide patient- and family-centered care, coordinate care across settings, and provide staff support.

End of Life Practice Issues: Withholding and Withdrawing Life-Sustaining Therapies

Limiting life-sustaining therapies in an ICU are becoming more common. It is estimated that withholding or withdrawing life support occurs in 67% to 84% of deaths in ICUs.[12] Generally, life-sustaining treatment is withdrawn when death is believed to be inevitable, despite aggressive interventions. The American College of Physicians (ACP)[13] supports the right of a competent patient to refuse life-sustaining and life-prolonging therapy. The ACP also notes that there is no moral difference between withholding and withdrawing therapy. In addition, critical care–related professional organizations have published position papers in support of the patient's autonomy regarding withholding and withdrawal decisions.[14]

If patients are unable to make treatment decisions, then these decisions must be made on the patient's behalf by surrogates or by the healthcare team. Optimally, patients' living wills or advance directives can provide the direction for decisions related to treatment withholding or withdrawal. However, completion rates of these documents remain low.[15] When surrogates are asked to participate in decision-making, it is recommended that a family-centered, shared decision-making approach be used. These approaches are recommended for major decisions involving limiting life-sustaining treatments, when survival is unlikely but possible, or when survival may come with significant impairment. Holding multidisciplinary family meetings is an effective way for families to arrive at decisions about the patient's goals of care and may help reduce the burden and distress they experience during this time. Because problems with decision-making and communication deficits around end of life care are still frequent sources of conflict in the ICU, having a guideline to follow for conducting family meetings may be helpful. Box 4.1 provides a list of steps for conducting a family meeting when the patient is unable to participate in the decision-making process. In addition, there are helpful mnemonic techniques that may improve the quality of the communication processes between ICU clinicians and family members during end of life care family meetings.[16]

Incorporating mnemonic communication approaches such as the ones listed in Table 4.1 or following the guidelines for conducting a family meeting has shown promise. For example, in a randomized controlled trial

Box 4.1 Conducting Intensive Care Unit Family Meetings

Prepare

Review the patient history and medical problems.

Coordinate who on the healthcare team will attend the meeting (should be multidisciplinary and include the attending MD, bedside RN, social worker, palliative care clinician(s), and other relevant healthcare team members).

Discuss goals of the meeting with the healthcare team.

Identify one team member as meeting leader.

Discuss which family members will be present.

Arrange a private, quiet location with seating for all.

Open the Meeting

Introduce all in attendance.

Establish the overall goal of the meeting, eliciting family goals as well.

Acknowledge that this is a difficult time and situation.

Set rules for the discussion (e.g., time frame for the meeting).

Elicit Family Understanding

Ask questions of family members and listen.

As they respond, think about:

What do they understand?
What do they believe will happen?
What are their emotions?

Identify Preferences for Decision-Making and Information Sharing

Identify how family members prefer to receive information and the level of detail they would like to receive.

Assess the family's preference for their role in decision-making (this can range from letting the physician decide to the family member assuming all responsibility for the decision).

Give Information

Give brief information (e.g., two points you really want them to understand) and allow time for family to ask questions.

Avoid medical jargon.

Do not talk too much or focus on technical matters.

Be transparent about uncertainty.

If patient is dying, be sure to use the words "death" or "dying."

(continued)

Box 4.1 (Continued)

Respond with Explicit Empathy to Family Emotions

Use the N-U-R-S-E mnemonic (see Table 4.1).

Don't fight, but rather join family statements of hopefulness, using wish statements (e.g., "I wish I could promise that things would get better. I hope he gets better soon too.").

See if the family can hope for the best but prepare for the worst.

After Giving Information, Ask about Concerns and Questions

"You just got a lot of information. What questions do you have?"

Elicit Patient and Family Values and Goals

Ask about the patient's goals, values, and previous discussion about end of life care.

Frame those wishes within the context of the current medical situation.

Avoid asking family, "What do you think we should do?" Instead, ask what they know about their loved one's preferences and maintain focus on the patient's perspective.

Identify pertinent cultural, ethnic, or religious beliefs that may influence communication, decision-making, family relationships, and concepts of death and dying.

Deal with Decisions that Need To Be Made

Make a recommendation based on patient and family goals.

Time-limited trials with clear endpoints may make sense in certain clinical situations.

Do not offer treatments that are inappropriate and when the burdens outweigh the benefits.

Do not speak of "withdrawing care" or "treatment." Affirm ongoing quality of care and reassure the family that care will never be withdrawn, but the focus of care may change.

Close the Meeting

Offer a brief summary of what was discussed.

Offer to answer questions and assure the family that the team is accessible.

Check in to make sure the family heard what you wanted them to hear.

Express appreciation and respect for the family.

Facilitate referrals to support services.

Make a clear follow-up plan, including scheduling the next family meeting.

Document and Debrief

Communicate the outcome of the meeting to the rest of the clinical team.

Document the meeting in the medical chart.

Table 4.1 Helpful Mnemonics for Family Meetings	
VALUE Technique[121]	**NURSE**[122]
V- Value and appreciate what the family has said	N- Name "You seem distressed [or angry or worried, etc.]"
A- Acknowledge family emotions	U- Understand "This must be very difficult for you."
L- Listen to the family	R- Respect "I can see how much you are trying to honor your Dad's wishes."
U- Understand the patient as a person through the family	S- Support "We will be there to help advise you."
E- Elicit family's concerns and questions	E- Explore "Tell me more about what you are thinking/feeling."

Sources: Curtis JR, Engelberg RA, Wenrich MD, et al. Studying communication about end of life care during the ICU family conference: development of a framework. *J Crit Care.* 2002;17(3):147–160; Pollak KI, Arnold RM, Jeffreys AS, et al. Oncologist communication about emotion during visits with patients with advanced cancer. *J Clin Oncol.* 2007;25(36):5748–5752.

comparing family members who received standard care to family members who received the VALUE intervention during their end of life care conference, researchers found that those family members who received the intervention had significantly lower symptom prevalence of post-traumatic stress disorder (PTSD), anxiety, and depression. Other investigators found that when using palliative care indicators, such as physician recommendation to withdraw life support and expressions of patients' wishes, and discussion of families' spiritual needs were reported, family member satisfaction with end of life decision-making was significantly higher. Other researchers have reported that the use of empathetic comments was associated with higher family satisfaction with communication. In another study, family members reported significant improvement in having their needs met when they participated in multidisciplinary family meetings conducted by palliative care nurses.[17]

ICU nurses can be integral in family meetings and improving surrogate decision-making. One investigator discussed five ways that the ICU nurse can assist families with surrogate decision-making: They can begin by preparing the family member for the role of being a surrogate. Next, they can organize regular meetings between the family and the multidisciplinary team. Then, once the meeting is scheduled, the nurse can prepare the family before each ICU family meeting on what to expect and what questions to ask. Fourth, they can provide emotional support to the family during the ICU meetings. Finally, they can be present for the family after the meeting. In one mixed-methods study assessing the effectiveness of using a nurse as a family support specialist, it was found that the intervention improved communication, improved discussion of the patient's values and preferences, and improved patient-centered care.[18]

Nelson and colleagues discussed the importance of ICU nurses being involved in family meetings. ICU nurses know the patient's condition, have knowledge of the family, and have a continuous presence at the bedside. In addition to this, they can provide continuity to the family as well as ensure that communication and decisions are consistent within the team.[19] However, this role is not always comfortable for the ICU nurse. Therefore, a group of researchers implemented an educational intervention to improve communication skills for ICU nurses to better prepare them for their role in interdisciplinary meetings. Nurses received training in key components of their role in ICU family meetings, strategies in dealing with strong emotions, and approaches to dealing with conflict. Nurses who attended this training reported more confidence in voicing concerns about patient care, being better able to initiate meetings, and having less anxiety in taking part in the meetings.

When a decision to forgo life-saving therapy is made in the ICU, there should be a concerted effort to evaluate all therapies, including blood products, hemodialysis, vasopressors, mechanical ventilation, total parenteral nutrition, antibiotics, intravenous fluids, and tube feedings, to assess whether these treatments could make a positive contribution to the patient's comfort. Withdrawal of therapies should be preceded by chart notations of do-not-resuscitate (DNR) orders and a note documenting the rationale for comfort care and removal of life support. There should be a clear plan of action and provision of information and support to the family. Adequate documentation of patient assessments, withdrawal decisions and plans, therapy withdrawal orders, and patient and family responses during and after withdrawal is essential.

However, there is considerable variability regarding physician recommendations and documentation of discussions with families regarding withdrawal of life support. In addition, there is considerable variability in the standardization around the process of withdrawing life support and decision-making. All of these inconsistencies may infer—rightly or wrongly—the lack of quality end of life and palliative care in the ICU.

Withdrawal of Ventilator Therapy with Consideration of Analgesic and Sedative Needs

It is important to understand the methods by which mechanical ventilation may be removed. Withdrawal of this treatment deserves the same clinical preparation as any other ICU procedure. The primary goal during this process should be to ensure that patients and family members are as comfortable as possible, both psychologically and physically. Two primary methods of mechanical ventilation removal exist: immediate extubation and terminal weaning (Table 4.2). Debates continue as to which of these methods is optimal for the patient, and often the method is determined according to the physician's, patient's, or family members' comfort levels. However, in one study, Szalados and colleagues reported a significant increase in family satisfaction with immediate extubation before death of their loved one in the ICU.[20]

Although there is considerable variability regarding the preferred approach to withdrawal, recommendations regarding specific procedures for withdrawal are available.[21,22] Box 4.2 presents a protocol for

Table 4.2 Methods of Mechanical Ventilation Withdrawal

Immediate Extubation	Terminal Weaning
Description	
Abrupt removal of the patient from ventilator assistance by extubation after suctioning (if necessary). Humidified air or oxygen is administered to prevent airway drying.	Physicians or other members of the ICU team (e.g., respiratory therapists, nurses) gradually withdraw ventilator assistance. This is done by decreasing the amount of inspired oxygen, decreasing the ventilator rate and mode, removal of positive end-expiratory pressure (PEEP), or a combination of these maneuvers. Usual time from ventilator to T-piece or extubation: 15–60 min.
Positive Aspects	
Patient free of technology; dying process less likely to be prolonged; intentions of the method are clear.	Allows titration of drugs to control symptoms; maintains airway for suctioning if necessary; patient does not develop upper airway obstruction; longer time between ventilator withdrawal and death; moral burden on family may be less because method appears less active.
Negative Aspects	
Noisy breathing, dyspnea may be distressful to patient/family.	May prolong dying; patient unable to communicate; machine between patient and family.
Time Course to Death	
Unpredictable. Usually shorter than with terminal weaning.	Unpredictable.

Sources: Truog RD, Campbell ML, Curtis JR, et al. Recommendations for end of life care in the intensive care unit: a consensus statement by the American College [corrected] of Critical Care Medicine. *Crit Care Med*. 2008;36(3):953–963; Billings JA. Humane terminal extubation reconsidered: the role for preemptive analgesia and sedation. *Crit Care Med*. 2012;40(2):625–630; Campbell ML. How to withdraw mechanical ventilation: a systematic review of the literature. *AACN Adv Crit Care*. 2007;18(4):397–403; quiz 344–395.

withdrawal of mechanical ventilation for the clinician's consideration that includes specific recommendations regarding use of analgesics and sedatives. Consensus guidelines on the provision of analgesia and sedation for dying ICU patients support the titration of analgesics and sedatives based on the patient's requests or observable signs indicative of pain or distress. The guidelines emphasize that no maximum dose of opioids or sedatives exists, especially considering that many ICU patients receive high doses of these drugs over their ICU course. Anticipatory dosing, as opposed to reactive dosing, is recommended by some to avoid patient discomfort and distress. Researchers surveying 143 nurses and 61 physicians on the usefulness of using a standardized order form for the withdrawal of life support found that the majority of nurses (84%) reported the form was helpful and were mostly satisfied with the sedation and mechanical ventilation sections. Almost all of the physicians (95%) reported that the form was helpful and were mostly satisfied with the sedation, mechanical ventilation, and death preparation sections.[23] Using a standardized order form is recommended; however, in a more recent study, only 12% of nurses reported

Box 4.2 A Protocol for the Withdrawal of Mechanical Ventilation

I. Anticipate and Prevent Distress

A. Review process in advance with patient (if awake), nurse, and family. Identify family goals during withdrawal (e.g., ability to communicate versus sedation). Arrange a time that allows the family to be present, if they wish.

B. Provide for special needs (e.g., clergy, bereavement counselor). Assess respiratory pattern on current level of respiratory support.

C. Use opioids and/or benzodiazepines* to control respiratory distress (i.e., respiratory rate >24 breaths per minute, use of accessory muscles, nasal flaring, >20% increase in heart rate or blood pressure, grimacing, clutching). In patients already receiving these agents, dosing should be guided by the current dose.

D. In the absence of distress, reduce intermittent mandatory ventilation (IMV) rate to less than 10 and reassess sedation.

E. Discontinue therapies not directed toward patient comfort:
   1. Stop neuromuscular blockade after opioids and/or benzodiazepines have been started or increased.[†]
   2. Discontinue laboratory tests, radiographs, and vital signs.
   3. Remove unnecessary tubes and restraints.
   4. Silence alarms and disconnect monitors.

II. Optimize Existing Function[**]

A. Administer breathing treatment, if indicated.

B. Suction out the mouth and hypopharynx. Endotracheal suctioning before withdrawal may or may not be advisable depending on patient distress and family perception. Consider atropine (1–2.5 mg by inhalation q6h), scopolamine (0.3–0.65 mg IV q4–6h), or glycopyrrolate (1–2 mg by inhalation q2–4h) for excessive secretions.

C. Place the patient at least 30 degrees upright, if possible.

III. Withdraw Assisted Ventilation[‡]

A. In general, changes should be made in the following order[§]:
   1. Eliminate positive end-expiratory pressure (PEEP).
   2. Reduce the fractional oxygen content of inspired air (FIO_2).
   3. Reduce or eliminate mandatory breaths.
   4. Reduce pressure support level.
   5. Place to flow-by or T-piece.
   6. Extubate to humidified air or oxygen.

B. Constant reevaluation for distress is mandatory. Treat distress with additional bolus doses of opioids and/or benzodiazepines equal to hourly drip rate and increase drip by 25% to 50%.

(continued)

Box 4.2 (Continued)

C. Observe for postwithdrawal distress, a medical emergency. A physician and nurse should be present during and immediately after extubation to assess the patient and to titrate medications. Morphine (5–10 mg IV q10 min) or fentanyl (100–250 µg IV q3–5 min) and/or midazolam (2–5 mg IV q7–10 min) or diazepam (5–10 mg IV q3–5 min) should be administered.

*Drug doses are difficult to specify because of the enormous variability in body weight and composition, previous exposure, and tolerance. In opioid-naïve patients, 2 to 20 mg morphine or 25 to 250 µg fentanyl, followed by an opioid infusion of one half of the loading dose per hour, is a reasonable initial dose.

†Usually the effects of neuromuscular blocking agents (NMBAs) can be reversed within a short period, but it may take days to weeks if patients have been receiving NMBAs chronically for management of ventilatory failure. Neuromuscular blockade masks signs of discomfort. Therefore, clinicians should feel that the patient has regained sufficient motor activity to demonstrate discomfort.

‡There is no one sequence applicable to all patients because their clinical situations are so variable. The pace of changes depends on patient comfort and may proceed as quickly as 5 to 15 minutes or, in an awake patient to be extubated, over several hours.

**These measures may be started earlier or before extubation if the patient is having excessive secretions.

§Patients who require high levels of ventilatory support may die after small adjustments such as reduction or elimination of PEEP or decrease in FiO_2 to 21%. In such patients, the physician should be present during and immediately after the change in therapy to assess the patient.

Sources: Kompanje EJ, van der Hoven B, Bakker J. Anticipation of distress after discontinuation of mechanical ventilation in the ICU at the end of life. *Intensive Care Med.* 2008;34(9):1593–1599; Szalados JE. Discontinuation of mechanical ventilation at end of life: the ethical and legal boundaries of physician conduct in termination of life support. *Crit Care Clin.* 2007;23(2):317–337, xi; Treece PD, Engelberg RA, Crowley L, et al. Evaluation of a standardized order form for the withdrawal of life support in the intensive care unit. *Crit Care Med.* 2004;32(5):1141–1148.

using standing orders to guide withdrawal of life support, and most (64%) were guided by individual physician's orders.[24]

It is important to provide comfort to dying patients who could experience pain and other distressing symptoms during withdrawal of mechanical ventilation. One group of investigators studying patients receiving morphine or morphine equivalents and benzodiazepines before mechanical ventilation withdrawal reported that these agents did not cause unintended harm and shorten survival time.[24] In another study, researchers found that increased dosages of morphine were actually associated with a longer time to death.[25] Therefore, clinicians should strive for symptom control at the end of life and ensure that comfort is maintained.

Patients should be withdrawn from neuromuscular blocking agents (NMBAs) before withdrawal from life support. The use of NMBAs (e.g., vecuronium) makes it almost impossible to assess patient comfort; although the patient appears comfortable, he or she may be experiencing pain, respiratory distress, or severe anxiety. The use of NMBAs prevents the struggling and gasping that may be associated with dying but not the patient's suffering.[26] The horror of such a death can only be imagined. The withdrawal of these agents may take considerable time for patients who have been receiving them chronically, and patients continue to have effects from lingering active metabolites.[27]

As mentioned earlier, research to guide the practice of ventilator withdrawal and factors associated with withdrawal is scant. One group of researchers assessed the process of withdrawal of life support in 88 ICU patients. They reported that 10% died after removal of vasopressors, 35% died after mechanical ventilation was withdrawn, and 55% died after the withdrawal of both mechanical ventilation and vasopressors.[24] Verkade and colleagues reviewed the charts of patients who had life-support treatments withdrawn to identify factors associated with this process. They found wide variability in practice; however, overall, forgoing active life-supporting treatment decisions was associated with older patient age, being admitted with medical versus surgical reasons, higher severity of illness scores, and severe central nervous system injury.[12] Finally, other investigators reported that most ICU clinicians used a stuttering withdrawal process (removing one treatment at a time) and that on average, removal of life-support treatment was prolonged (lasting longer than 1 day). In this study, they found that factors such as younger patient age, longer ICU stay, more life-sustaining interventions, and involvement of more decision-makers led to prolonged withdrawal.[28]

Regardless of the methods, factors, or processes used to withdraw life-sustaining therapies, the critical care nurse plays a major role during the decision and implementation of withdrawal of patients from mechanical ventilation. Increased nursing involvement can help provide optimal care to these patients and their families. Specifically, the nurse can be an active member at family meetings, where patient prognosis and goals of care are discussed. In addition, the nurse can ensure that a rationale for, and all elements of, the plan have been adequately discussed among the team, patient, and family. The nurse can ensure that adequate time is given to families and their support persons, such as clergy, to reach as good a resolution as possible. The family needs reassurance that they and the patient will not be left alone and that the patient will be kept comfortable with the use of medications and other measures. As discussed earlier, opioids, alone or in combination with benzodiazepines, are used during withdrawal to ensure that patients are provided the optimal degree of comfort.

Care for the Family of the Dying Intensive Care Unit Patient

Although the focus of care in many critical care areas is on the critically ill patient, nurses and other clinicians with family care skills realize that comprehensive patient care includes care of the patient's family. A family-centered approach to care is strongly supported by best practice recommendations, and this approach acknowledges a reciprocal and all-important relationship between the family and the critically ill patient. A change in one affects the other, and vice versa. Current research describes that an ICU experience for family members can be stressful (especially when their loved one dies in the ICU) and has been associated with symptoms of PTSD, anxiety, depression, and complicated grief, most recently termed *post–intensive care syndrome—family.*[29] Therefore, no discussion of palliative care in the ICU is complete without also discussing care of the dying patient's family. Family is defined here as any significant other who participates in the care and well-being of the patient.

The clinical course of any given critically ill, dying patient can vary tremendously, ranging from a rapid decline over several hours to a gradual decline over several days, weeks, and even months. Of course, the manner in which a family copes is also highly variable. Caring for families at any point along the dying trajectory, however, encompasses major aspects of access, information and support, and involvement in caregiving activities.

Access

A crucial aspect of family care is ensuring that the family can be with their critically ill loved one. Historically, critical care settings have severely restricted family access and discouraged lengthy family visitation. Commonly cited rationales to limiting family access include concerns regarding space limitations, patient stability, infection, rest, and privacy; the negative effect of visitation on the family; and clinicians' performance abilities. Some of these concerns have merit, whereas others, such as adverse patient-related issues and a negative effect on the family, have not been borne out in the research literature.[30]

Many ICUs around the world routinely limit visitors to two at any one time. Space limitations in critical care areas can be profound because most ICUs were designed for efficient use of life-saving machinery and staff and were not intended for end of life vigils by large, extended families. Ensuring that all interested family members have access to their loved one's bedside can present challenges to the often already narrow confines of the ICU. However, family members of dying loved ones should be allowed more liberal access (both in visiting time and in number of visitors allowed). Patients are confronting what may be the most difficult of life passages and therefore may need support from their family members. Researchers assessed 149 family members and 43 ICU workers regarding their perceptions of unrestricted visiting hours in the ICU. They reported that family members were more satisfied with this practice; however, ICU nurses and physicians stated moderate interruptions to patient care. Nurses reported a slight delay in organizing nursing care, and physicians reported greater unease when they were assessing the patient and perceived greater family stress, but they also perceived greater family trust.[31] Although healthcare professionals may feel that family visitation interferes with some aspects of patient care, the benefits far outweigh the risks.

Visitation of children should also be considered when a family member is dying. There is support for letting children visit the patient and become familiar with the care the patient is receiving and allowing them to understand what is going on. Visitation has the potential to help the child cope and gives the child a chance to say goodbye. If ICU clinicians account for the child's developmental status and properly prepare the child, then children can visit a critically ill family member in the ICU without ill effects.

There is a growing body of literature that supports family access to patients during invasive procedures and resuscitation. Facilitating family access during such times has come to be known as *facilitating family presence,* a practice supported by the Emergency Nurses Association[32] and the American College of Critical Care Medicine.[33] Several authors have reviewed the impact of family presence during procedures and have found that family members thought their presence benefitted their loved ones by being present to comfort and support them. Studies examining family satisfaction with family presence have yielded similar results,[32] and one study demonstrated no adverse psychological effects on the part of family members after the witnessed resuscitation, and as a matter of fact, found that families had lower symptoms of anxiety, depression, and PTSD.

Finally, caring for the critically ill, dying patient and his or her family can call forth feelings of failure for clinicians bent on finding a cure and force healthcare providers to reflect on their own mortality.[34] Even if family presence may be stressful for healthcare professionals and may not be fully embraced by ICU professionals, current literature reveals that family presence during resuscitation may help humanize the patient, improve communication, and help families with the grief process. Currently, it has been recommended that hospitals establish formal programs that allow immediate family members to be present during resuscitation. This program should include trained staff to support the family, assess the family for distress, educate the family regarding the process, and debrief after the process. The emotional burden for healthcare providers when providing palliative care is discussed later in this chapter.

Information and Support

Information has been identified as a crucial component in family coping and satisfaction in critical care settings. Support, in the form of clinicians' caring behaviors and interactions, is enormously influential in shaping the critical care experience for both patients and their families. In the context of caring for a critically ill, dying patient, however, nurses and physicians alike have reported high stress related to "death telling," or notifying family members of the patient's death or terminal prognosis. In general, very few healthcare providers feel they have the skills and knowledge necessary to counsel families effectively during this emotionally charged time. The ethical principle of honesty and truth-telling collides with the limits of knowing the truth precisely when there is clinical ambiguity and also collides with the suffering imposed on a family having to face the hard truth. Compassionate truth-telling requires dialogue and relationship, timing, and attunement, all of which are relational aspects that are frequently overlooked in the hectic pace of the ICU. Add patient, family, and healthcare provider culture to the equation, and one can readily understand why communication between involved parties is a less-than-perfect science.

Overall satisfaction with end of life care has been shown to be significantly associated with completeness of information received by the family member, support and care shown to the patient and family, consistency in staff, and satisfaction with the amount or level of healthcare received.

Family conferences have been used extensively as a means to improve communication between healthcare providers and family members, and the few studies that have investigated best practices in relation to the timing, content, and participants necessary for optimal communication during a family conference have shown improved satisfaction and lower emotional distress for family members. Encouraging family members to attend rounds has been shown to improve family satisfaction with the frequency of communication with physicians and the support with decision-making. In addition, diaries may help lower distress for family members. Researchers found that family members who recorded a diary during their loved one's ICU stay had lower levels of PTSD-related symptoms 12 months after the ICU experience.

Some hospitals have created interdisciplinary teams to improve communication and to help work with critically ill patients and their families in an effort to meet patients' and families' physical, informational, and psychosocial needs. Such teams usually include a nurse, physician, chaplain, and social worker. Working in concert with the nurses and physicians at the bedside, these interdisciplinary teams can more fully concentrate on end of life issues so that, theoretically, no patient or family needs go unmet during this time (Box 4.3)

Box 4.3 Case Study: Mrs. S

Palliative Critical Care? Using Intensive Care Unit Resources to Enhance Quality of Life in Serious Illness

Mrs. S had spent many years as a nurse providing primary care to underserved communities from Guatemala to Baltimore. She now lives on the coast with her husband and dog and enjoys swimming and hiking in the nearby national park. In 2010, she was diagnosed with multiple myeloma. She received several courses of chemotherapy, resulting in cardiomyopathy and renal failure. Mrs. S has spent 40 of the past 60 days in the hospital, receiving plasmapheresis and hemodialysis (HD) to prepare her for additional chemotherapy and possible stem cell transplantation.

August 15–17: Mrs. S presented to the hospital with several days of fatigue, worsening nausea, and decreased urine output. She was admitted to the oncology floor. Over the next three days, she received HD and plasmapheresis and was started on a new course of chemotherapy. Concern for tumor lysis syndrome necessitated aggressive intravenous (IV) hydration. Mrs. S began to develop lower extremity edema and crackles in her lung bases. Her blood pressure was becoming more tenuous, making it difficult to achieve desired fluid removal during HD.

August 18: Mrs. S had difficulty moving her legs, was unable to eat, and reported significant dyspnea. During HD, she began vomiting and became acutely hypotensive. She was transferred immediately to the medical-surgical intensive care unit (ICU). The oncology attending

(continued)

Box 4.3 (Continued)

physician informed Mrs. S that she would not be a candidate for stem cell transplantation. Nephrology ordered continuous renal replacement therapy (CRRT) to correct her electrolyte imbalances while preventing further fluid buildup.

That evening, Mrs. S had a lot on her mind, and her nurse Ron was ready to listen. Mrs. S revealed that she had made treatment decisions more for her loved ones than for herself. She had used this extra time to rebuild relationships with estranged family members and reflect on having accomplished so many of her life goals. Ron and Mrs. S rehearsed what it might be like to tell her husband that there would be no stem cell transplantation and, hopefully, no more chemotherapy. Mrs. S spoke of walking in the hills near her home and how her current state made that seem very far away. She talked about shopping at her local farm market and memorable family dinners. She hoped to return home for her last days, able to walk and eat. Ron pulled the ICU resident aside and passed along what Mrs. S had said, suggesting that a family meeting with all the teams and the palliative care service might be helpful.

August 19: The nephrologist stopped in to check on Mrs. S during breakfast, and they discussed her desire to shift to a palliative plan of care. In the last four days, Mrs. S had gained 20 pounds of water weight. In keeping with the new approach, the team began using CRRT to gently reverse her fluid excess. All services collaborated on moving IV medications and fluids to the oral route to facilitate the transition to home.

The attending physician from the palliative care service met with Mrs. S around lunchtime. She reported severe pain, primarily in her back and legs. With additional questioning, the physician determined that the pain appeared to have three main components: bone pain from a lesion in her spine, neuropathic pain emanating from her low back into all extremities, and discomfort due to edema now extending to her pelvis. He recommended starting daily methadone, with oxycodone for breakthrough pain. Dexamethasone was added as adjunctive therapy. He discussed options for additional neuropathy control, but Mrs. S was concerned that too many new medications might make her feel "woozy." She began taking senna to prevent constipation.

For Mrs. S, uncontrolled nausea permitted only small sips of water. The team started around-the-clock haloperidol, with sublingual lorazepam available for breakthrough nausea and vomiting. The new dexamethasone was expected to help as well.

When asked about her goals, Mrs. S had four that came to mind:

- Remove enough edema to allow her to walk
- Be able to swim near her home
- Spend time with her dog
- See her second grandchild, due to be born in one month

(continued)

Box 4.3 (Continued)

She requested palliative care service assistance in discussing expectations and plans with her husband. Mrs. S declined further chemotherapy and, at her instruction, a do-not-resuscitate order was placed in her chart.

Ron returned that night to the bedside, and he and Mrs. S worked hard together to take advantage of the new medications in managing her symptoms. They talked about the interdisciplinary family meeting scheduled for the next day and reviewed the four goals she had set for her remaining time.

August 20: The morning was brightened by a visit from a familiar face, the oncology social worker. Mrs. S updated her on the whirlwind events of the past few days and said, "I've made the right decision. It's OK to die."

Nephrology increased the CRRT fluid removal rate and discontinued all nonessential lab work. When the palliative care service physician examined Mrs. S, she was still experiencing severe back pain and nausea. He increased the around-the-clock dose of haloperidol and added promethazine. Scopolamine was offered; Mrs. S declined.

At 2 p.m., the family meeting was convened at the bedside. The team explained to Mr. S that there were no further curative therapies available for his wife. They offered that, under these circumstances, the current level of care could be refocused on maximizing comfort and quality of life. Mr. S was sad, but said he could see why his wife was ready to go home. The palliative care chaplain arranged to visit the next day to help Mrs. S write legacy letters to her grandchildren.

Mrs. S started the oral vasopressor midodrine to enable accelerated fluid removal with CRRT. She received the Sacrament of Healing from the visiting priest. Her spirits were much improved, and she expressed relief that "the end is in sight." When Ron returned for the night shift, he and Mrs. S worked with the ICU physicians to improve her pain control. Mrs. S spent several hours that night praying for the patient in crisis across the hall; she told Ron that, as a nurse herself, she wanted to help.

August 21: As morning approached, Mrs. S struggled with vomiting and was again unable to eat. When the interdisciplinary team met to formulate the day's plan of care, they decided to tackle nausea first. The oncology service ordered daily high-dose dexamethasone and another run of plasmapheresis. The palliative care service added dronabinol to the plan.

Over the course of three days in the ICU, CRRT had removed 6 liters of fluid. Mrs. S had continuous cardiac and arterial blood pressure monitoring, making it possible to safely deliver this therapy. Lower extremity edema had improved to 2+, and her lungs were clear nearly to the bases. Nephrology ordered a further increase in the hourly CRRT fluid removal rate.

Mrs. S shared with the team that, for the first time, she believed she would make it home. To each person entering her room, she expressed

(continued)

Box 4.1 (Continued)

her thanks and challenged them to keep pushing her. She and the chaplain took advantage of some down time to reflect and work together on letters to her grandchildren. During the night, her one-on-one nursing care continued—fine-tuning doses and frequencies of medications so that Mrs. S would have the best possible regimen on which to discharge home.

August 22: Mrs. S's nausea was under control, and her diet was advanced to "as tolerated." She felt well enough to enjoy a long-anticipated bit of black coffee for breakfast! The day got even better when her nurse brought a walker to her room and assisted her out of bed. Together they walked to the end of the ICU, where an enormous picture window faces the Golden Gate Bridge and the sea. Standing there with her nurse, Mrs. S could almost see home.

Later that day, the teams met with Mrs. S and her family. "We're ready to get her home—this is our window of opportunity," Mr. S noted. The oncology and palliative care social workers set up home hospice referral, had durable medical equipment delivered, and located a pharmacy near the tiny town where the family lived.

August 23: When the palliative care team visited Mrs. S, she was in her bedside chair, watching the news and breathing room air. CRRT had been discontinued a few hours earlier. The attending physician completed the Physician Orders for Life Sustaining Treatment (POLST), reflecting Mrs. S's request not to be resuscitated or receive artificial nutrition and hydration. The hospice and hospital providers coordinated next steps for symptom management and psychosocial support. Ron stopped in to say goodbye. A little while later, Mrs. S went home—to walk, swim, and relax with her dog. She died a week later, in her own bed, on her own terms.

Case courtesy of Kathleen Turner, RN, BSN, CHPN, CCRN-CMC, Adult Medical-Surgical ICU, University of California San Francisco Medical Center, San Francisco, CA.

Finally, because feelings of grief in surviving family members are still commonly unresolved one year after a loved one's death, many critical care units have organized bereavement follow-up programs. These programs typically involve contacting the surviving family (by telephone or mail) monthly for some period of time and at the one-year anniversary of their loved one's death. In addition to remembering and supporting the family, these programs have also been shown to help healthcare providers cope with the loss as well. Another suggestion that may be helpful to family members is that the ICU staff can hold memorial services twice a year for family and friends of the patient to reconnect with the critical care staff. During this service, names of those who have died in the past 6 months are read. A reception is held afterward that gives everyone, especially the staff, an opportunity to reflect on their work and to honor the people they have served.

References

1. Angus DC, Barnato AE, Linde-Zwirble WT, et al. Use of intensive care at the end of life in the United States: an epidemiologic study. *Crit Care Med.* 2004;32(3):638–643.

2. Wunsch H, Linde-Zwirble WT, Harrison DA, et al. Use of intensive care services during terminal hospitalizations in England and the United States. *Am J Respir Crit Care Med.* 2009;180(9):875–880.

3. Teno JM, Gozalo PL, Bynum JP, et al. Change in end of life care for Medicare beneficiaries: site of death, place of care, and healthcare transitions in 2000, 2005, and 2009. *JAMA.* 2013;309(5):470–477.

4. Miesfeldt S, Murray K, Lucas L, et al. Association of age, gender, and race with intensity of end of life care for Medicare beneficiaries with cancer. *J Palliat Med.* 2012;15(5):548–554.

5. Levin TT, Moreno B, Silvester W, Kissane DW. End of life communication in the intensive care unit. *Gen Hosp Psychiatry.* 2010;32(4):433–442.

6. Puntillo KA, Arai S, Cohen NH, et al. Symptoms experienced by intensive care unit patients at high risk of dying. *Crit Care Med.* 2010;38(11): 2155–2160.

7. The SUPPORT Principal Investigators. A controlled trial to improve care for seriously ill hospitalized patients. The Study to Understand Prognoses and Preferences for Outcomes and Risks of Treatments (SUPPORT). *JAMA.* 1995;274(20):1591–1598.

8. Delgado-Guay MO, Parsons HA, et al. Symptom distress, interventions, and outcomes of intensive care unit cancer patients referred to a palliative care consult team. *Cancer.* 2009;115(2):437–445.

9. Spronk PE, Kuiper AV, Rommes JH, et al. The practice of and documentation on withholding and withdrawing life support: a retrospective study in two Dutch intensive care units. *Anesth Analg.* 2009;109(3):841–846.

10. Gay EB, Pronovost PJ, Bassett RD, Nelson JE. The intensive care unit family meeting: making it happen. *J Crit Care.* 2009;24(4):629.e1–12.

11. White DB, Curtis JR, Wolf LE, et al. Life support for patients without a surrogate decision maker: who decides? *Ann Intern Med.* 2007;147(1):34–40.

12. Verkade MA, Epker JL, Nieuwenhoff MD, et al. Withdrawal of life-sustaining treatment in a mixed intensive care unit: most common in patients with catastrophic brain injury. *Neurocrit Care.* 2012;16(1):130–135.

13. Snyder L. American College of Physicians Ethics Manual: sixth edition. *Ann Intern Med.* 2012;156(1 Pt 2):73–104.

14. American Association of Critical Care Nurses (AACN). *Position Statement: Withholding and/or Withdrawing Life-Sustaining Treatment.* Newport Beach, CA: AACN; 1999.

15. Kumar A, Aronow WS, Alexa M, et al. Prevalence of use of advance directives, healthcare proxy, legal guardian, and living will in 512 patients hospitalized in a cardiac care unit/intensive care unit in 2 community hospitals. *Arch Med Sci.* 2010;6(2):188–191.

16. Spinello IM. End of life care in ICU: a practical guide. *J Intensive Care Med.* 2011;26(5):295–303.

17. Hudson P, Thomas T, Quinn K, Aranda S. Family meetings in palliative care: are they effective? *Palliat Med.* 2009;23(2):150–157.

18. White DB, Cua SM, Walk R, et al. Nurse-led intervention to improve surrogate decision making for patients with advanced critical illness. *Am J Crit Care*. 2012;21(6):396–409.

19. Nelson JE, Cortez TB, Curtis JR, et al. Integrating palliative care in the ICU: the nurse in a leading role. *J Hospice Palliat Nurs*. 2011;13(2):89–94.

20. Szalados JE. Discontinuation of mechanical ventilation at end of life: the ethical and legal boundaries of physician conduct in termination of life support. *Crit Care Clin*. 2007;23(2):317–337, xi.

21. Curtis JR. Caring for patients with critical illness and their families: the value of the integrated clinical team. *Respir Care*. 2008;53(4):480–487.

22. Curtis JR, Treece PD, Nielsen EL, et al. Integrating palliative and critical care: evaluation of a quality-improvement intervention. *Am J Respir Crit Care Med*. 2008;178(3):269–275.

23. Treece PD, Engelberg RA, Crowley L, et al. Evaluation of a standardized order form for the withdrawal of life support in the intensive care unit. *Crit Care Med*. 2004;32(5):1141–1148.

24. Kirchhoff KT, Kowalkowski JA. Current practices for withdrawal of life support in intensive care units. *Am J Crit Care*. 2010;19(6):532–541, quiz 542.

25. Mazer MA, Alligood CM, Wu Q. The infusion of opioids during terminal withdrawal of mechanical ventilation in the medical intensive care unit. *J Pain Symptom Manage*. 2011;42(1):44–51.

26. Truog RD, Brock DW, White DB. Should patients receive general anesthesia prior to extubation at the end of life? *Crit Care Med*. 2012;40(2):631–633.

27. Truog RD, Burns JP, Mitchell C, et al. Pharmacologic paralysis and withdrawal of mechanical ventilation at the end of life. *N Engl J Med*. 2000;342(7):508–511.

28. Gerstel E, Engelberg RA, Koepsell T, Curtis JR. Duration of withdrawal of life support in the intensive care unit and association with family satisfaction. *Am J Respir Crit Care Med*. 2008;178(8):798–804.

29. Davidson JE, Jones C, Bienvenu OJ. Family response to critical illness: postintensive care syndrome-family. *Crit Care Med*. 2012;40(2):618–624.

30. Whitton S, Pittiglio LI. Critical care open visiting hours. *Crit Care Nurs Q*. 2011;34(4):361–366.

31. Garrouste-Orgeas M, Philippart F, Timsit JF, et al. Perceptions of a 24-hour visiting policy in the intensive care unit. *Crit Care Med*. 2008;36(1):30–35.

32. Egging D, Crowley M, Arruda T, et al. Emergency nursing resource: family presence during invasive procedures and resuscitation in the emergency department. *J Emerg Nurs*. 2011;37(5):469–473.

33. Davidson JE, Powers K, Hedayat KM, et al. Clinical practice guidelines for support of the family in the patient-centered intensive care unit: American College of Critical Care Medicine Task Force 2004-2005. *Crit Care Med*. 2007;35(2):605–622.

34. McMillen RE. End of life decisions: nurses perceptions, feelings and experiences. *Intensive Crit Care Nurs*. 2008;24(4):251–259.

Chapter 5

Palliative Care Nursing in the Outpatient Setting

Pamela Stitzlein Davies

The vast majority of healthcare in the United States is provided in ambulatory care clinics. Although palliative care (PC) has become incorporated into most major acute care hospitals, it is still relatively novel in the outpatient (OP) clinic, especially in noncancer settings.[1] Meier and Beresford describe the provision of PC in the outpatient setting as the "new frontier."[2] The American Society of Clinical Oncologists (ASCO) has a goal of providing PC as a routine part of comprehensive cancer care for all patients by 2020, and specifically states that PC should be available in all of the settings that care is received, including OP clinics.[3] In 2014, ASCO, in conjunction with the American Academy of Hospice and Palliative Medicine (AAHPM), launched a three-year collaborative with 25 practice sites, designed to improve the quality of PC provided in the OP setting.[4] In addition, the Center to Advance Palliative Care (CAPC) has developed a website to promote and improve OP PC.[5] Thus, the field of OP PC is anticipated to expand significantly in this decade.

Patients are living longer and with greater disabilities than ever before. In addition to advanced cancer, other terminal diseases managed in ambulatory care include end-stage heart failure, advanced cirrhosis, renal failure, and terminal neurologic disorders such as advanced dementia. Primary and specialty care providers are central in the care of these advanced illnesses, but they receive minimal training on end of life (EOL) care and are challenged to find the time to address these essential issues.[6] Nurses and advance practice nurses (APNs), with their extensive psychosocial training, and in collaboration with a multidisciplinary team, play an important role in helping ambulatory clinic patients and caregivers navigate concerns that arise as EOL approaches. This chapter addresses the provision of PC in the adult OP setting, with a focus on the role of nurses and APNs.

Advantages and Challenges Faced in the Outpatient Setting

The OP setting is ideal for providing PC because the pace is less crisis-driven than inpatient care and typically benefits from long-term trusting relationships that form between the patient, caregiver, and medical team over months and years. These factors permit dialogues on advance care planning to be held over a series of visits, allowing the patient to absorb small "doses" of information at a time and to discuss these options with loved ones in the comfort of their home environment. Other advantages of providing PC in the OP setting are listed in Box 5.1.

Challenges faced in the OP setting are described in Box 5.2. Some of these challenges are common to PC teams in any setting, such as receiving late referrals (when a patient is actively dying) and funding issues. Other issues are specific to the OP setting, such as coordinating OP PC visits with the primary team's appointments. A unique issue faced by some OP PC programs is referrals for management of chronic pain not related to the primary diagnosis (e.g., chronic low back pain requiring ongoing moderately high-dose opioid therapy in a patient with a curable leukemia) or for ongoing management of chronic pain in a cancer survivor years after completion of therapy. Because most PC programs focus on patients with terminal illness, long-term management of complex chronic pain problems may be beyond the parameters of what the PC team can offer. However, in some institutions, the chronic pain clinic is combined with the PC clinic and has the expertise and manpower to manage these cases on a chronic basis.

Box 5.1 Advantages of Providing Palliative Care in the Outpatient Setting

- Early involvement by the PC team in pain and symptom management helps build relationships with patients and caregivers; this can foster communication during times of stress or crisis.

- The OP setting is less crisis-driven, allowing patients and caregivers to confer about advance care planning in "little doses," months or years before decisions are needed.

- Continuity of care between the inpatient PC and OP PC services allows for seamless PC involvement when the patient is admitted or discharged.

- OP PC may result in fewer emergency department visits and fewer admissions or readmissions.

- PC results in earlier recognition and treatment of depression and anxiety in patients and caregivers.

- PC results in improved quality-of-life ratings in patients, despite continued physical decline.

- PC fosters less "overaggressive" chemotherapy in the final weeks of life.

- PC promotes earlier hospice referral, resulting in improved quality at end of life.

- PC is associated with a potential for survival benefit.

Box 5.2 Challenges Faced when Providing Palliative Care in the Outpatient Setting

- Patients may feel abandoned or believe that a referral to PC means the clinician is "giving up" on them.
- Clinician's misunderstanding of the PC role may result in late referrals to the PC service, when a hospice referral is more appropriate (e.g., the patient is actively dying).
- Providing excellent communication and seamless coordination of care with the primary team takes extra time and effort on the part of the PC team.
- Scheduling challenges occur when trying to consolidate patient appointments by coordinating PC appointments on the same day as the primary clinician's appointment.
  - PC appointments scheduled in an OP oncology infusion center may be challenging because of administration of sedating pre-medications, such as diphenhydramine, making the visit impossible because the patient is sedated. In addition, lack of privacy may limit visits in this area.
- Lack of funding for clinician and support staff salaries
- Lack of availability of clinic examination room space
- Challenge in providing staffing for 24/7 telephone availability by the PC team
- Determining who "owns" patient symptom management issues. For example, who manages chemotherapy-induced nausea? Who titrates the pain medicines and prescribes the opioid renewals?
  - A special issue in outpatient oncology is which team (oncologist or PC) is responsible for addressing a new pain problem. Depending on the individual setting, most PC teams in a consultant or collaborative role will defer the workup of new pain syndromes to the oncologist because the pain may be due to progression of malignancy resulting in a change of chemotherapy or initiation of radiotherapy.
- Although some OP PC programs may be able to accept all referrals, most will need to define and limit the type of consultations accepted owing to staffing limitations. If scheduled, the OP PC team might elect to limit their involvement to only a few visits. For example:
  - Referrals of patients who have moderate symptom burden from chronic disease but who are not in advanced state of illness, with anticipated life expectancy of decades
  - Management of chronic pain issues that are not related to the advanced illness in the cancer survivor with anticipated long-term management needs or in the patient with active substance use

Primary, Secondary, and Tertiary Palliative Care

Primary palliative care describes the role that every nurse, APN, and other medical provider plays in recognizing and addressing PC needs in ambulatory settings. Also referred to as "generalist" PC, this includes skill sets such as basic pain and symptom management and EOL discussions and related paperwork. Because PC resources are limited, referrals should focus on patients with complex needs who require specialty consultation.[7] In addition, the majority of community oncology care is provided in settings that lack PC resources. Thus, the clinic team members act in a front-line role for the provision of the majority of PC needs. For example, when a patient arrives in pulmonary clinic for a post-hospitalization visit after a chronic obstructive pulmonary disease (COPD) exacerbation, his nurse may inquire whether any discussions occurred regarding advance directives and code status during the recent inpatient stay. Often, patients receive paperwork from the inpatient social worker related to such discussions but do not complete it. The clinic nurse can help them finalize the forms during the clinic visit or notify the social worker to assist. Another example of primary palliative care in symptom management is when the oncology nurse reminds patients to use a bowel management plan when taking opioids for cancer pain. Ambulatory care nurses also play a key role in providing education and support in the decision to transition to hospice care. Ongoing learning is needed to keep nurses and clinicians up to date on basic palliative care skills.[6] The essential role of the clinic nurse in addressing PC needs cannot be overemphasized: these concepts are at the very heart of nursing. In other words, every nurse should be providing primary palliative care on an ongoing basis.

Secondary palliative care refers to the formal involvement of PC specialists to assist with more complex cases.[3] Problems addressed may relate to complicated pain and symptom management, maladaptive coping and distress, or assistance with particularly challenging EOL situations. *Tertiary palliative care* describes major PC programs with a focus on research and teaching to advance the specialty and may include a PC physician and advanced practice registered nurse (APRN) fellowship programs.[8]

As OP PC expands into nononcology fields, such as cardiology or neurology, PC specialists must become familiar with specific PC topics that arise in various fields. Some topics are common to all fields, such as advance care planning; other topics are unique to a specialty, such as the decision to stop dialysis. Box 5.3 lists some of these topics.

Models of Care

Three basic models exist in the delivery of OP PC: collaborative, consultative, and medical home.[9] The *collaborative* (also known as embedded, integrated, or concurrent) model is the most popular style found in the

Box 5.3 Sample Topics Addressed in Outpatient Palliative Care by Specialty

- All Sites
  - Pain management
  - Symptom management
  - Psychosocial spiritual distress, coping with serious illness
    - Recognizing and addressing existential distress that contributes to the pain experience
    - Assisting the primary team in working with "challenging patients," such as those with significant psychopathology (schizophrenia, personality disorder) that creates disruptions in care or "staff splitting"
  - Treatment decisions, future planning
    - Goals of care discussions
    - Completion of advance directives, durable power of attorney for healthcare, do-not-resuscitate orders
  - Caregiver issues
    - Coping, stress management, education, respite needs
  - Decision and timing of referral to hospice
  - Requests for hastened death
- Oncology
  - Decision-making related to stopping chemotherapy and other treatments. This is usually required to enroll in hospice.
  - Decision to move forward with a hematopoietic cell transplantation when anticipated outcome is poor
  - Moral distress experienced by infusion nurses related to ongoing transfusion of blood products (a scarce resource) for transfusion-refractory anemia or thrombocytopenia (e.g., an end-stage acute myelogenous leukemia patient, with no active bleeding, not on treatment, who is receiving ongoing platelet transfusions three times a week, despite a minimal rise in the post-transfusion platelet count)
- Neurology
  - Discussions regarding initiation or discontinuation of tube feedings or ventilator in end-stage dementia, amyotrophic lateral sclerosis, or multiple sclerosis
- Nephrology
  - Decision not to initiate or to discontinue dialysis
  - Issues around inclusion or removal from kidney transplant list
- Cardiology
  - Complex decisions regarding initiation or discontinuation of left ventricular assist devices
  - Turning off automatic internal cardiac defibrillator
  - Issues around inclusion or removal from heart transplant list

(continued)

Box 5.3 (Continued)

- Pulmonary
  - Discussion about do-not-intubate orders
  - Issues around inclusion or removal from lung transplant list
- Hepatology
  - Issues around inclusion or removal from liver transplant list
  - Patient distress related to personal behaviors that may have contributed to the development of hepatocellular carcinoma (e.g., use of intravenous drugs decades prior, leading to development of hepatitis C, leading to higher risk for hepatocellular carcinoma)
- Primary Care/Geriatrics
  - Care decisions in debility, failure to thrive, dementia, including placement in skilled nursing facilities
  - Assisting the primary care provider in explaining or confirming specialty recommendations (e.g., why treatment of breast cancer is not recommended in a frail 92-year-old woman with severe dementia)
  - Assisting the primary care provider with management of complex hospice cases, especially if the specialty provider (oncology, cardiology or neurology) has signed off the case

outpatient setting. In this model, the PC team takes the lead in managing certain aspects of care, such as pain and symptoms, distress, or decision-making, thus allowing the clinician (oncologist, cardiologist) to focus on the overall management of the patient. In the collaborative model, the PC team institutes its own recommendations, including writing prescriptions, and follows patients on an ongoing basis, often in coordination with its clinic follow-up visit. Advantages of this model are combining "the best of both worlds," with specialists from both fields contributing to care and working together to improve quality of life (QOL) in distinct, yet complementary, roles. Embedded clinics create the opportunity for a shared visit with the clinician, thus improving communication and coordination of care. This model is usually more convenient for the patient, especially if PC visits are held on the same day and location as his or her other clinic appointment. However, it creates special challenges for the scheduling of PC visits to accomplish that coordination. For optimal success in this model, the PC team must consider themselves *diplomats*, with ongoing efforts to foster a good relationship with the referring clinician, striving for flexibility to work within the framework of that clinician's practice style.[10] For example, some clinicians may object to the PC team discussing questions about prognosis before they have addressed that subject themselves.

In the *consultative* model, the PC provider evaluates patients and forwards management recommendations to the team for their implementation. The PC team does not write prescriptions and does not implement the recommended plan of care. In addition, PC does not typically follow patients on an ongoing basis. Unfortunately, this model may suffer from lack of follow through on the PC recommendations. Rabow found that a low percentage of patients had the plan of care implemented, when using a consultative model in a primary care clinic to address pain and depression, among other issues.[11] However, patients seen under this model could potentially benefit if the structure and goals of the visit were specifically defined. For example, when a nurse meets with a patient to discuss goals of care and advance planning, that single visit fulfills the PC intervention. Research is needed to further define methods to make this model work well.

The final model of care is the *medical home model* (defined in the literature as the "primary palliative care" model, which is different than the same term discussed earlier). In this model, the PC team functions as the "medical home" or "primary care provider" and addresses all aspects of the patient's care: from management of the life-limiting illness, such as end-stage liver disease, to other chronic conditions, such as hypertension and osteoarthritis.[12] This model integrates PC into primary care and is an excellent option for medically underserved populations and for patients who are not eligible for, or elect not to pursue, specialized treatments such as dialysis or chemotherapy. The clinician must have a broad knowledge base and access to specialists for formal or informal consultation. In many ways, this model is comparable to services traditionally provided for decades by general practitioners.

Key Studies in Outpatient Palliative Care

Several important trials have shown the advantage of using PC in the OP setting. The most notable is that reported by Temel and colleagues[13] examining the effect of providing early PC to patients recently diagnosed with metastatic non–small cell lung cancer (NSCLC), which typically has a prognosis of less than a year. This was a nonblinded, randomized controlled study of 151 patients, with 74 patients receiving standard care and 77 patients receiving embedded PC in addition to standard care. The PC team, consisting of six physicians and one nurse practitioner, met with patients within 12 weeks of diagnosis and saw them monthly until death. The visits focused on symptom management, psychosocial distress, goals of care, and treatment decisions. The findings, which received wide publicity, showed that patients in the PC arm lived 30% longer than the control group (11.6 vs. 8.9 months) and reported better QOL with fewer symptoms of depression, despite receiving less aggressive treatment at EOL and earlier hospice enrollment.

In a pilot study led by an APRN, Prince-Paul and colleagues[14] studied the impact of PC on adults with advanced cancer in an OP oncology clinic. Fifty-two patients received usual care, and 49 received usual care plus PC provided in a collaborative model. More than 50% of the patients received chemotherapy during the study. PC visits focused on pain and symptom management; medicine education; psychological, social, and spiritual support; and discussions about EOL preparation. Patients were followed for five months. Findings revealed that those in the PC arm were 84% less likely to be hospitalized and 25 times more likely to be alive at four months compared with the usual-care group. In addition, higher scores on social well-being scales resulted in fewer hospitalizations and lower mortality. The authors concluded that the provision of PC by an APRN in the oncology setting is beneficial and that the provision of emotional support and active presence by the PC nurse may explain some of that benefit.

Bakitas and colleagues[15] randomized 322 subjects with advanced cancer to either usual care or usual care with PC, under the study name of Project ENABLE (Educate, Nurture, Advise, Before Life Ends). This APRN-led study involved four structured psychoeducational sessions, followed by monthly telephone calls. Educational topics included patient activation, self-management, self-advocacy, and communication skills to use with their oncologist. The intervention group showed improvement in QOL and mood scores, demonstrating the ability of nurse-led education to empower the cancer patient.

Murphy and colleagues[12] examined the healthcare use of 147 patients enrolled in a *medical home PC* model compared with the 12-month period before enrollment. Patients received care for a variety of life-limiting illnesses, such as cancer, heart failure, COPD, dementia, and end-stage renal disease, in addition to management of other primary care issues. Most participants from this county "safety-net" academic medical center struggled with mental illness, substance use, or homelessness. The results of the chart review showed a 27% reduction in emergency department visits and a 20% reduction in hospitalizations after enrollment in the PC program. This confirmed the findings of the pilot study in this population by Owens and colleagues[16] and again demonstrated the success of APRNs in providing both primary care and PC to patients with life-limiting illness.

Muir and colleagues[10] examined the benefits of an embedded PC team in a private oncology practice. This study focused on provider satisfaction and time saved by the oncologist, in addition to quality care outcomes. PC involvement resulted in a 21% reduction in symptom burden, increased oncologist satisfaction, and saved an estimated 170 minutes of oncologist time for each new referral seen by the PC team.

Practical Details in Providing Outpatient Palliative Care

Many questions arise when developing or expanding an OP PC program. This section addresses common issues in implementation, with a focus on oncology clinics because most of the literature exists in the oncology setting.

Referrals to the Outpatient Palliative Care Team

Referrals to OP PC depend on multiple factors unique to the individual provider, clinic milieu, and organizational setting. In a survey of 12 OP PC centers, oncologists initiated 76% of the referrals, and 23% came from the inpatient PC team.[17] Other factors include the needs and expertise of the referring clinician (oncologist, nephrologist), access to supportive care services in the referring clinic (social work), percentage of patients in the practice with complex needs, and availability of PC clinicians. Close physical proximity to the referring clinician appears to play a major role in generating consults. However, each clinician has a different personal threshold regarding who would benefit most from employing the PC team. Triggers for referral may be based on diagnosis, symptoms, or psychosocial factors.[17] Box 5.4 lists common criteria for a consult to OP PC.

Establishing an ongoing referral base is important when building and maintaining a PC OP practice because most patients die within weeks or months of an initial PC visit. The embedded PC practice model creates the most referrals, especially if the PC practitioner can see a new consult soon after, or even concurrently with, the referring clinician to assist with "bad news" discussions or complex symptom management. Participating in multidisciplinary clinic rounds (tumor board or heart failure clinic) can increase PC visibility and generate referrals. PC rounds in which complex patient

---

Box 5.4 Sample Referral Criteria to Outpatient Palliative Care

Patient/Symptom Characteristics

- Limited treatment options, such as very advanced hepatocellular carcinoma
- Diagnosis of highly fatal malignancies, such as metastatic non–small cell lung cancer, pancreatic cancer, or esophageal cancer
- Anticipated poor outcomes, such as in elderly patients with acute myelogenous leukemia or patients undergoing "high-risk" stem cell transplantation
- Diagnosis of end-stage cardiac, pulmonary, renal, or hepatic disease
- Poorly controlled pain or other symptoms
- Declining functional level (e.g., Eastern Clinical Oncology Group [ECOG] score of 3 or 4, or Palliative Performance Scale of ≤50)
- Frequent emergency department visits or hospitalizations
- Enrollment in a phase 1 chemotherapy trial

Psychosocial Circumstances

- High levels of psychological, social, or spiritual/existential distress
- Poor social support
- Inability to engage in advance care planning discussions
- Family discord in decision-making
- Requests for hastened death

Other

- Staff issues including moral distress and compassion fatigue

cases are discussed and educational programs on complex symptom management are other options that may act to generate referrals.

In our setting, any clinician may send a referral to OP PC. In addition to the oncologist, clinic policy allows nurses, social workers, physical therapists, and chaplains to generate a consult. Infusion center nurses are a great source of referrals. These nurses form close relationships with patients over months, sometimes years, of chemotherapy and frequently have in-depth discussions about coping with cancer. If the patient experiences worsening symptoms or distress that is not well managed at the "primary PC" level (e.g., nurse or oncologist level), the nurse may refer to PC for expert assistance without first obtaining the oncologist's approval. Some oncologists initially expressed concern regarding this policy because they are in charge of the overall care and well-being of the patient and were concerned that PC involvement might cause the patient to "lose hope." In response, the PC team made significant efforts to maintain positive relationships and close communication with the oncologists, with a focus on methods the PC team can use to assist and decrease their workload. In addition, research findings supporting positive outcomes of PC involvement were reviewed on a formal and informal basis.

Finally, in our clinical setting, patients may self-refer to PC, with information on PC provided on the clinic website and brochures. Clinic volunteers who assist in the waiting room and often hear stories of suffering from the patient are encouraged to offer a PC brochure and instruct that they may self-refer by calling the PC telephone. Referrals also come from family members or leaders of community cancer support groups. In these cases, the PC nurse or coordinator will contact the patient directly to describe the PC service and confirm their interest in scheduling an appointment. On occasion, PC will see a caregiver alone, without the patient present, to discuss EOL planning. However, verbal permission is first obtained from the patient.

Organizational Recommendations for Palliative Care Referral

In 2012, the ASCO issued a Provisional Clinical Opinion recommending that all patients with metastatic NSCLC be offered PC, along with standard oncologic treatment, based on the findings of Temel and colleagues.[13] In addition, the National Comprehensive Cancer Network (NCCN) guidelines on PC listed a broad range of referral criteria.[18] Although such widely inclusive referral criteria are ideal, they are probably not realistic for most organizations because of limitations in PC resources. A strategy is needed to identify those most in need of a referral to secondary- and tertiary-level PC specialists. For that reason, use of algorithms is becoming more common in the inpatient and OP settings.[19]

Glare and collegues[20] developed a screening tool for PC referral in an OP gastrointestinal (GI) oncology clinic based on the NCCN PC guidelines. This one-page instrument assigned zero to 13 possible points for five items: metastatic or locally advanced disease (two points); ECOG score (zero to four points); serious complication of advanced cancer (hypercalcemia, cachexia—one point); serious comorbid disease (heart failure, cirrhosis—one point); and five specific PC problems (uncontrolled symptoms, high levels of distress, decision-making, specific request for referral, complex decision-making/goals of care—one point each). The clinic nurse screened 119 patients over a three-week period. Depending on the threshold used, 7% to 17% of patients would be eligible for PC consultation. The authors further determined that a score of five or higher had the best predictive value and would trigger a PC consult in 13% of the GI oncology clinic population. However, the screening process took three to five minutes per patient, resulting in a burdensome one to two hours of nursing time per clinic day. The authors suggest that prepopulating the instrument with diagnosis from the electronic medical record (EMR) and having the patient self-report on symptoms and distress could reduce the screening time. Of course, this requires the EMR to have accurate diagnostic information (e.g., "metastatic colon cancer," not just "colon cancer") and serious comorbidities (such as stage 3 congestive heart failure) provided in the problem list. The authors suggested screening at the initial visit, after hospitalization, and every 6 months. Interestingly, the clinic nurse indicated that *all* patients met the NCCN standards for a referral to PC, further emphasizing the need to prioritize primary PC from secondary or tertiary care.

Screening New Patient Referrals

When receiving a PC referral, it is helpful to ascertain several key points.

- First, *what is the purpose of the consult?* If the referral only indicates "palliative care, evaluate and treat," it is helpful to speak with the referring team to ask what specifically triggered the referral request for this patient. Are there signs of maladaptive coping with progressive disease? Is the caregiver insisting on aggressive treatment when the patient seems to want to stop chemotherapy? Is the patient experiencing ongoing severe symptoms, despite standard treatment? A few minutes spent clarifying the purpose of the consult can help the PC team to better understand the situation and focus the visit.

- Second, *what is the urgency of the consult?* Should the consult be scheduled immediately, or can the initial PC visit be held until the patient returns for the next chemotherapy visit in 3 weeks? An important observation is that what is deemed urgent by the referring source (oncologist, neurologist) may not appear urgent to the PC team or even to the patient.[15] For example, the patient may call the nurse and express high levels of distress, asking for any kind of help as soon possible, but then decline to schedule a next-day appointment with the PC team, preferring to wait a few weeks.

- Third, *are the patient and caregiver aware of the consult?* Even if they are aware, it is surprising how many patients and caregivers perceive the PC referral as abandonment, saying to the scheduler: "I guess this is how Dr. Jones is telling me he's giving up on me." Therefore, the scheduler has an important and delicate task when setting up the initial visit to explain the purpose of PC involvement. If there appears to be any confusion or hesitation, the referring team should be notified and asked to assist with communication regarding the PC consult.

The wait time from referral to first PC appointment is ideally less than 1 week, with urgent consults scheduled even sooner.[1] This may be a challenge for many programs because of provider staffing limitations. If the PC physician's schedule is filled and an urgent same-day consult cannot be accommodated, the PC nurse may assist by assessing the patient's needs. The nurse then discusses the case with either the primary provider (oncologist) or the PC provider and follows up with the patient by telephone, if needed. The PC provider is then scheduled to see the patient as soon as possible.

Maintaining a Good Relationship with the Referring Physician

Success in providing OP PC in the collaborative model requires maintenance of positive relationships with the referring specialty physician (oncologist, neurologist, cardiologist), the nurse, and other team members. It may be helpful to think of the physician as the "customer" and PC as the service the customer is "buying." Close communication and a respectful approach are key, along with negotiation of "who does what" in patient care.[14] For example, opioids for pain management and cough are prescribed by the PC service, but the oncologist prescribes 3 days of steroids to reduce chemotherapy-induced nausea with each cycle. It is important for the PC team members to respect this provider's specialized skills and acknowledge that they have known this particular patient for years, and in some cases even decades. In addition, it is helpful to recognize that the physician, as the "captain of the ship," may feel threatened when referrals to PC are generated by another source, especially if the physician believes that everything is stable. To smooth this process, our team sends an e-mail to the oncologist noting that a referral was received, who it was from (infusion nurse, inpatient PC provider), and what services were requested (e.g., coping with recent news of disease progression, management of symptoms) and asking for contact if there are any questions or concerns about PC involvement in the patient's care. After each visit, the oncologist and team nurse are updated on the patient's status through an EMR note. An e-mail with additional information is sent, if there are particular points to highlight, for example, to inform the oncologist that the patient was started on an antidepressant for anxiety management. Direct personal communication with the oncologist is always attempted if there are major issues, such as the patient's request to stop chemotherapy and enroll in hospice. Although this coordination of care takes a significant amount of time, it is immensely helpful in keeping relationships positive and assures future referrals.

Because there are many drug interactions with chemotherapy, it is incumbent on the PC team to consult with the team pharmacist or pharmaceutical references before writing new prescriptions. This will prevent serious drug interactions (e.g., methadone, ondansetron, and citalopram all cause QT prolongation) but may also highlight the potential inactivation of the anticancer therapy by certain drugs (e.g., paroxetine on tamoxifen.) To prevent creating problems and more work for the primary team, it is essential to check potential interactions before a prescription is written.

Team Members Providing Outpatient Palliative Care

The OP PC team may range from a part-time PC nurse in the oncology clinic to a fully staffed interdisciplinary palliative care team consulting five full days per week in a range of OP clinics. In a recent survey of 20 OP PC programs in a variety of practice settings, 19 clinics used physicians, 10 sites had APRNs, 14 had registered nurses, and 12 had a social worker.[1] The full time equivalent (FTE) staffing varied widely, ranging from a sole physician working 0.25 FTE to an academic cancer center with 5 FTE, which included two physicians, two APRNs and one registered nurse. For physicians, in particular, it is common practice to have multiple providers filling a position. For example, one academic oncology site has six physicians, each working 0.1 FTE, for a total physician FTE of 0.6. This may create challenges in continuity of care and team cohesiveness. Two additional surveys showed that nurses and APRNs typically represent the majority of staff appointments, with nurses the most common employees (0.9 to 1.7 FTE), followed by APRNs (0.7 to 0.9 FTE), social workers (0.7 to 0.8 FTE), and physicians (0.3 to 0.6 FTE).[17,21]

Other PC team members may include chaplaincy, pharmacy, nutrition, and rehabilitation medicine staff such as physical, occupational, and speech therapists. The essential role of chaplaincy in addressing existential and spiritual distress cannot be overstated. Reports of "pain" in the dying patient may arise from *spiritual pain* and require the specialized input of a chaplain. Access to a board-certified chaplain is fundamental to the success of an OP PC team.[20,21] Finally, Bookbinder and colleagues[22] noted that inclusion of a social worker in their study resulted in 100% completion of advance directives, in addition to providing psychosocial support.

Components of the Palliative Care Visit

Patients dealing with advanced illness have many needs affecting multiple domains of suffering. Determining what issues to address at the initial OP PC visit depends on the needs identified by the patient, the stated purpose of the consult (e.g., symptom management, assistance with goals of care), and the specialty of the PC clinician (social worker vs. pain specialist). To assess the patient's perspective on priority of issues, inpatient PC subjects were asked, "What bothers you most?" Categories of initial patient response were: physical distress, 44%; emotional, spiritual, existential, or nonspecific distress, 16%; relationships, 15%; concerns about death and dying, 15%; loss of function or normalcy, 12%; distress about being in the hospital, 11%; distress with medical providers or treatment, 9%; miscellaneous, 15% (more than one category was stated by some).[23]

To further define the components of a PC visit, Yoong and colleagues[24] investigated 20 randomly selected patients with lung cancer from the

Temel study,[13] analyzing PC and oncologist chart notes in detail. Based on panel analysis of PC notes, the following key elements of a PC visit were identified:

- Relationship and rapport building
- Symptom evaluation and management
- Coping strategies
- Illness understanding
- Discussing cancer treatments
- End of life planning
- Engaging family members

This study was particularly interesting because the detailed analysis found that the PC team focused initially on building relationship and illness understanding, whereas discussions about resuscitation preferences and hospice became more prevalent at a later time, after "clinical turning points" occurred such as disease progression.

In another study of OP PC, components of a Supportive Care Team intervention were assessed in a nonrandomized study of 278 patients, with advanced GI or ovarian cancer.[24] These components were identified as:

- Assessment of patient symptoms and distress and the social and spiritual concerns of the patient and caregiver
- Documentation of the plan of care in the EMR
- Provision of support for patient and caregiver needs
- Advance care planning discussions, as early as possible
- Minimum of monthly contact with patient
- Telephone availability daily
- Regular meetings with the oncologist to review and coordinate patient care
- Referral to home care or hospice, as appropriate

Von Roenn and Temel[25] identified five domains of care for PC visits:

- Physical symptoms
- Spiritual care
- Assistance with practical needs
- EOL care
- Support for decision-making

Finally, in our practice, three major domains guide the framework of practice: providing pain and symptom management, addressing psychosocial spiritual needs, and assisting with future planning for those faced with a serious illness, such as advance directives and timing of hospice enrollment. Patients are told, "Dr. Smith asked me to talk to you about your sleep problems, but I'd also like to know what you feel is most important for us to talk about today." If multiple issues are identified, the patient is asked to prioritize the top two items. In this way, the primary needs of the patient and those of the referring provider are addressed at the initial visit, with additional issues deferred to follow-up visits.

Length of Palliative Care Visits

The literature indicates a variety of visit lengths for OP PC, but a key consensus is that providing palliative care takes time, and quality care cannot be rushed.[25] Initial visits are typically 60 minutes, and follow-up visits are 30 to 60 minutes. However, many clinicians discover that returning patients often need as much time as the initial visits. Disease progression leads to an increase in the number and intensity of symptoms, news of progressive illness creates worsening distress, and EOL decision-making becomes more of a priority. In addition to the patient visits, a significant amount of PC time is spent in coordinating care with the specialty clinician (oncologist, pulmonologist), which may take as long as five to 15 minutes before and after each visit. As noted previously, such coordination helps to "keep everyone on the same page," assists with role delineation (e.g., who is writing the prescriptions for antiemetics), and keeps the relationship with the specialty provider strong.

In a subanalysis of the Temel study,[13] Jacobsen and colleagues[26] described six components of the OP PC visit. These components, along with the median and range of time spent at the initial visit, include:

- Symptom management (median 20 minutes, range zero to 75 minutes)
- Patient and caregiver coping with a life-threatening illness (median 15 minutes, range zero to 78 minutes)
- Illness understanding and education (median 10 minutes, range zero to 35 minutes)
- Decision-making (median zero minutes, range zero to 20 minutes)
- Care planning and referrals (median zero minutes, range zero 20 minutes)

Initial visits lasted a median of 55 minutes, with a range of 20 to 120 minutes. Not surprisingly, patients who rated low on quality of life, as measured by the Functional Assessment of Cancer Therapy—General (FACT-G) scale, required longer visits; and higher depression scores, as measured by the Patient Health Questionnaire (PHQ-9), predicted greater time spent on symptom management.[26] A Canadian study found that initial visits with a nurse and physician team took 90 to 120 minutes.[27] Another paper reported combined nurse practitioner and social worker initial visits were scheduled for 90 minutes.[2] At our clinic, we schedule initial visits for 60 to 90 minutes and return visits for 30 to 60 minutes depending on the anticipated length of time needed.

Measures Used in Clinic Visits

A wide variety of instruments are used to gather research data in the OP PC clinic visits. These fall into the major categories of functional scales, global symptom scales, pain scales, psychological and social measures, spiritual assessment, and QOL. However, it is less clear what measures are typically used in nonresearch, everyday clinical practice. Consideration should be given to using a formal assessment tool because one study found a 10-fold increase in reported symptoms with a formal tool compared with open-ended questioning by a provider. Similarly, I have found that use of clinical (nonresearch) tools significantly helps with symptom reporting. Two scales are used regularly in practice: the Edmonton Symptom Assessment Scale (ESAS) and the Brief Pain Inventory, Short Form (BPI-SF). The ESAS is a commonly used PC clinical tool that lists a variety of symptoms (pain, fatigue, appetite, anxiety), rated on a zero to 10 scale, with zero being no symptom and 10 being the worst symptom possible. The BPI-SF includes a body diagram for indicating pain location, with zero to 10 pain intensity rating scales for worst, least, average, and current pain; word descriptors of pain; and pain interference scales such as activity, mood, and sleep. Additionally, the PHQ-9, a brief nine-item depression screening survey, is used when significant depression is suspected.

Another brief clinical screening tool is the Distress Thermometer. This is a simple drawing of a vertical thermometer with a zero to 10 numerical rating scale labeled "no distress" at zero, "moderate distress" at five, and "extreme distress" at 10. A score of five or higher indicates that a consult to specialized psychosocial support is needed. This tool has been validated in multiple OP clinical settings and is recommended by NCCN as a quick measure of distress.

Funding the Outpatient Palliative Care Program

A practical aspect of clinic viability is the need to secure sources of ongoing funding. Billing revenue is insufficient for OP PC programs to become self-sustaining, especially for APRN-led clinics, because of lower reimbursement rates for nonphysician providers. Most clinics require institutional support to survive. Other sources of funding include philanthropy, private foundation support, and research grants.

Management by telephone is a major aspect of the provision of OP PC (see "Telephone Support"). Although these calls can make the difference between a patient's remaining comfortably at home rather than making a trip to the emergency department, such cost avoidance data are difficult to capture. Thus, in some settings, the PC team may be challenged to find unique methods to demonstrate to leadership that the PC nurse role makes a difference and is not simply another salary expenditure. This may be easier to demonstrate in a managed care setting. More research is needed to support the cost benefit of OP PC, especially for non-reimbursable costs.

Telephone Support

As noted previously, support by telephone is a key function of the PC nurse. This role may start before the initial visit, when the PC nurse calls to confirm the upcoming appointment and answer any questions from the patient or caregiver. It is not unusual for patients to indicate that they do not understand why they have an appointment with PC. A simple description that works well is: "PC provides an extra layer of support for you and your family. We specialize in helping with pain, symptoms, and coping with the stress of serious illness." It is important to emphasize that the patient's doctor (oncologist, neurologist, cardiologist) will remain in charge of the patient's overall care and that the PC team will provide expert assistance (unless the patient is seen in the medical home PC model).

A telephone check a few days after the initial visit is beneficial to assess whether patients are following the treatment plan and if the problem is better, worse, or unchanged. The call also functions as a reminder that the PC team is now involved in their care. It is particularly important to follow up by telephone after a patient receives bad news (e.g., disease progression) or a referral to hospice because such events can lead to great distress, loneliness, and a sense of abandonment. An expression of concern for the patient and caregiver's welfare is always appropriate and may aid in distress management.

Telephone contact may be useful in other ways. Some patients seem more amenable to addressing the scary "what if" questions via a telephone conversation than in person. For example, "What is it going to be like when I die? Will I suffer?" Caregivers may have questions that concern them greatly but that they do not want to ask in front of the patient, such as, "What do I do if he starts to bleed?" "Will he choke to death?" Patients should be encouraged to call if there are questions or concerns and be reassured that they are not "bothering" the team in any way when they call. Often, we tell patients "we would much rather that you call, even if you think it is a small problem, because we can help before it becomes a bigger problem."

And finally, a condolence call or note card sent a few days or weeks after the patient's death allows an opportunity to say a final goodbye. Family members can be encouraged to make use of hospice bereavement services to assist them in their grief. Such calls or notes are an important gesture and may assist with closure, both for the bereaved and for the PC team who provided care.

Prescriptions

Renewal of opioid and other Schedule II drug prescriptions (oxycodone, morphine, fentanyl, methylphenidate) is a special concern for nonhospice patients because these drugs cannot be "called in" to a local pharmacy. Because many patients come from a long distance away, they are asked to notify the PC team a week before the opioid medicine runs out to allow time to mail the prescription and fill it at a local pharmacy. Writing Schedule II opioid prescriptions, completing insurance paperwork for prescription prior approvals, and enrolling patients in the Risk Evaluation Management Strategy (REMS) program (for transmucosal fentanyl prescriptions) can be very time consuming for providers and may be a reason that some of the consults are sent to the PC service.

Patient Education

An important aspect of nursing is patient education. This is especially true in the PC setting, when patients are often too fatigued and caregivers too stressed to remember information. Simple and clearly written instructions are essential to achieve compliance with the plan of care and thus to better control symptoms. A copy is given to the team nurse to communicate the PC interventions and also aids in "keeping everyone on the same page" in the collaborative care model. A follow-up call in a few days by the PC nurse can further refine patient education, check whether the instructions were instituted (e.g., increased dose of pain medicine), and answer questions. Preprinted instruction sheets on commonly reviewed PC topics, such as pharmacologic and nonpharmacologic pain management, constipation prevention and management, sleep hygiene, relaxation and coping techniques, and websites with helpful information, will streamline the provision of information for the patient.

Communication Skills for the Nurse

Excellent communication skills are at the heart of PC nursing.[9] These skills, which include both verbal and nonverbal communication, can be intentionally learned; they are not an "innate" ability possessed by a select few. However, becoming proficient takes time and practice. For clinic nurses interested in providing primary palliative care, learning a few basic techniques will enhance their ability to understand and address patient and caregiver needs. For nurses at the secondary and tertiary level of PC practice, expertise in complex communication practices, including conducting family meetings, is a key proficiency.

In a document titled *Peaceful Death: Recommended Competencies and Curricular Guidelines for End of Life Nursing Care,*[28] training is recommended for nurses to become competent in EOL communication. These skills are important in all fields of nursing, particularly oncology, nephrology, and geriatrics, in which a significant number of deaths would be anticipated. Box 5.5 lists several techniques for interacting with patients and caregivers in the OP setting. Two helpful resources are provided by Back and colleagues[29] and Malloy and colleagues.[6] Nurses are encouraged to attend an End of Life Nursing Education Consortium (ELNEC) course to gain further knowledge in EOL communication and other skills.[30]

Talking to Patients and Caregivers About Prognosis

Ideally, physicians, APRNs, nurses, and other team members are able to provide realistic prognosis estimates that are clearly communicated to patients and caregivers, with appropriate and timely referrals to hospice. However, it is not uncommon for nurses to hesitate when speaking about prognosis for a variety of reasons. In a survey of 174 experienced hospital nurses, five categories were identified that created obstacles for nurses to speak to patients and family about prognosis and hospice referral.[31] These

Box 5.5 Palliative Care Communication Skills

- "Ask, Tell, Ask"
  - Ask patients a series of questions to elucidate their understanding of the situation, their hopes and concerns, and how they prefer to receive information.
  - Offer to share information ("Would it be okay if I shared some thoughts on this decision?").
  - Follow up with more questions on the patients' response and perspective.
- NURSE: This acronym describes methods of acknowledging and responding to patient or caregiver emotion.
  - Naming: Name the emotion you are observing ("It sounds like you are upset with the news of the scan results you got today.")
  - Understanding: Seek to gain an understanding of the impact of the emotion ("This must be very disappointing.")
  - Respecting: Show empathy by use of verbal or nonverbal acknowledgement of the patient's emotion, or praise for their coping skills (with an expression of concern—"I have always been impressed with your efforts to follow the medical instructions exactly. I know you have done everything possible to fight the cancer.")
  - Supporting: Share a statement of partnership and support for the future because patients fear abandonment. Make sure your statement is something realistic and truthful ("I will be here to support you on the road ahead.")
  - Exploring: Explore emotional cues further ("You mentioned this was the worst thing that could ever have happened to you. I'd like to understand a bit more of what you mean by that. Can you tell me a little more?).
- Silence is golden.
  - The use of silence is a key communication technique. Although it may seem like "nothing is happening," this is an important time that allows the patient and caregiver to collect their thoughts, get in touch with deep emotions, and process suffering.
  - It is appropriate to consider the use of silence when patients or caregivers become tearful, when they appear to be processing information or formulating questions, or when they seem reticent to speak.
  - Use of silence should be accompanied by an active and attentive presence by the nurse (this is not a time to check the clock or catch up on charting.).
  - Periods of silence may last five to 30 seconds or longer. This takes practice to become comfortable! Start out by allowing short periods of silence lasting five to seven seconds, then build the length, as appropriate.
  - Empathetic presence through silence can be a form of *witness* to the suffering that is being endured and is thus therapeutic.

(continued)

Box 5.5 (Continued)

- Use communication continuers.
  - Examples include: "Tell me more," "it sounds like this has been very difficult," or "help me to understand why that upset you so much."
  - Be aware of your body language and strive for "open" nonverbal communication by body turned toward the patient, appropriate eye contact, concerned expression, and keeping your arms and legs uncrossed.
  - When the patient is crying, after a period of silence, ask, "Can you tell me about the tears?"
- Recognize conversation terminators used by the patient or caregiver.
  - "I'm getting tired." "Maybe we could talk about this some other time."
  - Nonverbal cues (crossed arms, sighing, looking at watch, tapping a pencil). You can address this by simply asking, "I get the sense that you are ready to end the visit at this point?" Or, "Your wife still has several questions on her list, but you look like you're getting tired. Would you prefer to rest in the waiting room while we finish talking?"
- Perceiving the unspoken message.
  - Expert nurses excel in "hearing" the unspoken message. This involves paying attention to potential messages in order to uncover concerns in the cultural, spiritual, or psychological domains.
  - For example, a patient question about the probability of future worsening pain may actually mean, "I'm afraid I'm going to die in terrible pain!"
  - Issues involving worsening sleep may uncover untreated anxiety or existential distress.
  - Asking the same questions repeatedly may also point to untreated depression and anxiety, as well as high levels of fear and distress about the future.
- Guided narrative in palliative care. These questions will help the PC team understand the patient's and caregiver's perspectives.*
  - "What is your understanding of your current situation?"
  - "What are you hoping for?"
  - "What concerns you the most?"
  - "What gives you strength to get through every day?"
  - "What do you value most in life?"
  - "Is religion or spirituality important to you?" "Are you at peace?"
  - "What are your experiences with serious illness or death?" "What do you know about hospice care?"
  - "What else would you like the team to know about you so that we can provide you with the best care?"

*Adapted with permission from Farber S, Farber A. The respectful death model: difficult conversations at the end of life. In: Katz RS, Johnson TA, eds. *When Professionals Weep: Emotional and Countertransference Responses in End of Life Care. Series in Death, Dying, and Bereavement.* New York, NY: Routledge; 2006:221–237.

included: (1) unwillingness of patient or family to accept the prognosis or hospice referral; (2) sudden death or change in patient status, which prevented communication; (3) belief of physician hesitance or perception that physicians did not feel it was the nurse's role to speak about prognosis; (4) nurses' discomfort in speaking about death, or feeling they were too busy to address the topic; (5) nurses' desire to maintain hope in the patient and family and desire to prevent them from getting upset. Although this was an inpatient study, it is likely that these issues also affect nurses in the ambulatory care setting.

Nurses may face a dilemma when a patient or caregiver directly asks about prognosis because some oncologists and other specialty physicians may object to a nurse (or even a PC physician) attempting to answer this question. However, the literature indicates that oncologists, as well as primary care providers, are not particularly good at estimating prognosis and tend to be overly optimistic. When there are clear signs and symptoms that the patient is moving into a terminal phase, the nurse may feel a moral obligation to speak up in order to allow appropriate preparation for death but may also fear that this may impede the relationship with the oncologist, if the oncologist objects to the nurse having such conversations. One method of resolving this dilemma is to use a communication technique called "Ask, Tell, Ask." A technique that addresses emotion is the acronym NURSE: naming, understanding, respecting, supporting, exploring. Both of these techniques are explained in more detail in Box 5.5.

Using these methods, the nurse can elucidate the patient's knowledge about prognosis, without stating something that the physician may find objectionable. Patients often have an "inner knowing" that their time is short and death is approaching. By using open-ended questions, the nurse can explore the patient's perception in a supportive manner. Box 5.5 has an example of this technique. In the example, the euphemistic statement, "I'm worried that your time might be shorter than we hope," allows the nurse to address her moral dilemma by expressing her concerns about shorter prognosis, without explicitly contradicting what the oncologist told the patient (or the patient's *perception* of what he or she was told) about prognosis. As the oncologist becomes more comfortable and trusting of the nurse's judgment and communication skills, it is hoped that moral dilemmas such as this example occur less frequently.

Maintaining Hope in the Face of Advanced Illness

As part of the human experience, we all need hope, especially when faced with a serious and life-limiting illness. The nurse may be concerned that such discussions may "destroy hope." However, hope can be maintained, even at EOL, through "redefining" what is hoped for. As disease progresses, and death approaches, our hopes change. Fanslow-Brunjes describes this process as the *Four Stages of Hope*: (1) hope for a cure, (2) hope for treatment that works, (3) hope for prolongation of life, and (4) hope for a peaceful death.[32] The skillful nurse can facilitate this transition of hope through the various stages by focusing on what *can* be done to help the patient. It is always essential to remember that "just being there," with empathetic, nonverbal communication, provides support and comfort to the patient and family members as they face an uncertain future. The impact of *presence* in the face of suffering is meaningful and cannot be overlooked. Nurses can excel in this simple but extremely powerful intervention that can engender hope and reduce suffering.

Staff Education

Providing staff education regarding the PC role is a common mission of the PC nurse, even if it is not part of the formal job description. Education on a formal or informal basis will help the clinic nurses and providers grow in their ability to provide primary palliative care of symptom management, distress management, coping with advanced illness, and preparation for EOL. For example, the PC nurse gives an in-service to infusion center nurses on tips for supporting patients experiencing high levels of distress. Or, an oncology physician assistant asks for a curbside consult with the PC APRN regarding appropriateness for the use of methylnaltrexone in a patient with severe opioid-induced constipation.

Common informal education involves reassuring providers that PC involvement does not preclude use of antineoplastic therapies. For example, an oncologist may state, "he's not ready for palliative care yet," in reference to a patient with stage IV non–small cell lung cancer who is starting second-line therapy and was referred to PC by an infusion nurse for symptom management. This provides an excellent opportunity for the PC team to explain the benefits of PC involvement and dispel myths. It is unfortunate that many oncologists still equate palliative care with hospice. This is an important distinction because most hospice agencies require patients to stop chemotherapy in order to enroll. By explaining the broader scope of PC compared with hospice and explaining that involvement of the PC team does not preclude the use of chemotherapy or other aggressive treatments, the conduit may be opened for additional referrals from that oncologist. Another example is a self-referral from a patient who faces a difficult but potentially curable treatment, such as a stem cell transplantation for acute myelogenous leukemia. The hematologist may say, "We're planning to cure this patient! We don't need PC!" Clear explanations that the goal of PC involvement is to "add an extra layer of support" to the patient and caregiver as they move through the aggressive transplant process with the goal of a cure and reassurance that the transplant team will be kept abreast of all discussions should reduce concerns.

Other opportunities for staff education may involve boundary setting regarding tasks that can be handled at the primary palliative care level. An example would be an urgent request for the PC team to immediately enroll a new patient in hospice, despite the absence of pressing physical or emotional needs. On further questioning, the team nurse indicated a lack of knowledge about how to enroll someone in hospice and presumed the PC team took care of this for all patients in the clinic. The PC APRN respectfully explained that this is the responsibility of the team nurse in this facility. Education was then provided regarding the necessary paperwork to collect and assistance with locating the appropriate hospice agency.

Similarly, a physician paged the OP PC APRN asking for completion of a do-not-resuscitate (DNR) order on the Physician Orders for Life-Sustaining Treatment (POLST). Inquiry revealed no complex issues with this patient; however, the oncology fellow was unfamiliar and uncomfortable with this process. Discussing a DNR decision is an essential aspect of medical care, of which every provider should have a basic working knowledge. Therefore, the PC APRN provided brief coaching, then offered to join the visit while the fellow explained the form to the patient and assisted with DNR decision-making. Thus, the provider gained skill in this important task, and the PC team was available to address more complex or unusual situations that might arise in the future.

Conclusion

This is an exciting time of momentum in the field of OP PC. As the discipline grows and matures in the oncology arena, attention is turning toward expanding PC into clinics with large numbers of terminally ill patients, such as cardiology, nephrology, neurology, and geriatrics. With the mandate of the Patient Protection and Affordable Care Act of 2010, the role of OP PC in preventing emergency department visits, hospital admission, and readmission will become more imperative.

Because there are more patients than can be seen by the limited PC resources, screening methods or algorithms should be used to identify those who are in the greatest need of referral. For the remainder, clinicians and nurses must learn the skills for providing primary palliative care in the OP setting.

Nurses play an important role in the provision of OP PC, with research showing that nurses or APRNs provide the bulk of staffing in these settings. Nursing skills are well adapted to the issues commonly addressed by the PC team (Box 5.6). With additional training in programs such as ELNEC, every nurse can become a palliative care nurse.

Box 5.6 Case Study: Bob

Bob is a 67-year-old white man with metastatic renal cell carcinoma (RCC). He underwent left nephrectomy when initially diagnosed and has subsequently been on a variety of chemotherapy and biologic agents over the past few years. He moved to town a year ago from the Midwest to be closer to family but then sought experimental treatment at a major cancer center on the East Coast for a period of 4 months, which depleted much of his savings. He lives alone, but his son and his family live nearby. Bob's oncologist, Dr. J, referred him to OP PC for pain management. He presents to the initial outpatient palliative care visit accompanied by his daughter-in-law, Gina. His chief complaint is severe and uncontrolled pain, despite transdermal fentanyl 200 mcg/hour every 72 hours; and oxycodone 5-mg tablets, ordered one to two every four hours as needed for pain, but he is taking 20 tablets per day (100 mg per day) with minimal relief. The most recent scan shows massive tumor invasion of the pelvis destroying a portion of the right iliac crest, involving the right iliopsoas muscle, with implants invading the sciatic nerve. Bob has declined to take anticonvulsives or antidepressants for neuropathic pain and has also deferred radiation therapy.

As the initial visit proceeded, it became apparent that Bob had a unique and "prickly" personality. He had a strong need to manage the pace and direction of the visit, frequently holding up his hands to halt discussion so that he could take meticulous notes. (He declined an offer to audiotape the visit for future reference.) Bob highly values having control of all medical decisions; he must thoroughly and carefully research each possible option for cancer treatment and pain management before he will agree to consider it, to such a degree that it appears to be interfering with his anticancer treatment and his comfort. Gina is clearly frustrated with this process, explaining that it usually takes weeks or even months for him to make any decision and is the reason he has not yet started radiation therapy for pain control.

The advanced practice registered nurse (APRN) discusses options with Bob and recommends the addition of gabapentin for neuropathic pain, short-term dexamethasone for rapid pain control, and initiation of the radiotherapy previously ordered. Because Bob does not want to change his opioid dose, she suggests switching to oxycodone 15-mg tablet to decrease the number of short-acting opioid tablets he is taking each day. After extensive discussion and negotiation, Bob eventually agrees to start the radiation therapy and to take dexamethasone 4 mg daily for two weeks. He does not agree to a trial of gabapentin and does not want any changes in his opioid pill strength. The initial visit took over an hour, with the entire conversation involving negotiation of pain control options.

The PC team followed Bob every 2 to 4 weeks, coordinating visits with his oncologist appointments. The patient slowly began to trust the APRN, especially as his pain started to improve. After many visits, and with extensive negotiation, he agreed to start gabapentin for neuropathic

(continued)

pain and eventually also agreed to add duloxetine for neuropathic pain and mood. Despite these strategies, his pain remained severe. The APRN started introducing the concept of existential distress as a potential significant component of Bob's pain experience. Although he did not accept that psychological or spiritual issues had any impact on him, his relationship with the APRN had developed to the point that he was willing to listen to the concept. He also appeared more comfortable and relaxed during the visits, taking notes, but no longer insisting on controlling each visit.

Bob remained strongly optimistic that he had many more years to live. However, after becoming intensely frightened during a pain crisis that led to a three-night hospital stay, he initiated discussions about his eventual demise. (He refused to see the inpatient PC team, indicating that he wanted to talk about these issues only with his OP PC APRN, after discharge.) Bob asked detailed questions about the dying process, wanting to know what he needed to do to prepare himself. Durable power of attorney for healthcare and do-not-resuscitate paperwork was completed. Hospice enrollment was discussed, and Bob agreed to meet with the hospice providers but subsequently cancelled the appointment and did not return their calls.

Several weeks later, Bob called the PC team, complaining of severe pain, but refused the PC APRN's advice to come into the clinic or emergency department for evaluation. After multiple telephone discussions between the hospice providers and Bob and Gina over the next three days, Bob ultimately agreed to enroll in hospice. However, this triggered significant worsening of his anxiety, and the compulsive component of his personality emerged once again. He was reluctant to follow through on the hospice team's advice for pain management and called the OP PC APRN repeatedly, despite her ongoing reassurance that she was working closely with the hospice nurse to manage his pain. Gina also called the OP PC team several times each week, in exasperation, wondering how to best help Bob. He was still living alone and declined to allow a hired caregiver in the home, despite having total immobility of the right leg, repeated falls, and difficulty managing his medications. He refused to see the hospice social worker or chaplain, despite high anxiety and distress levels.

By this time, he was on high-dose methadone for cancer pain, with high doses of hydromorphone for breakthrough pain. He remained in severe pain and appeared to be developing opioid-induced hyperalgesia. The OP PC APRN called Bob and recommended admission to the inpatient hospice center to initiate a ketamine infusion. She also reminded him of the option for an intrathecal block, which had been discussed multiple times over the months, but Bob had always declined it because of the associated risk for leg weakness. After several days of consideration, while experiencing progressive and severe pain, Bob agreed to be transported to the inpatient hospice unit, where he stayed for 12 days. A ketamine

Box 5.6 (Continued)

infusion and hydromorphone patient-controlled analgesia were started, resulting in much improvement in pain control. He was converted to oral ketamine 30 mg three times daily, and methadone was decreased to 30 mg three times daily. While Bob was an inpatient, the hospice social worker and chaplain were able to make explorations into existential distress as a contributor to his pain experience. Significant issues were uncovered and addressed, and Bob appeared to be more at peace. Once the pain was better controlled, he was discharged to home and agreed to hire a caregiver. This was a special time of bonding for Bob and his son, daughter-in-law, and two young granddaughters. He was delighted with the infectious joy of the children and would let them paint his toenails, play silly games, and snuggle with him in his hospice bed while he napped.

Bob did surprisingly well for six weeks, then fell and broke his pelvis, resulting in new, severe pain. It took three days for him to agree to hospital admission. He was deeply disappointed when told by the orthopedic surgeon that the fracture could not be repaired because of extensive bone erosion. Realizing he would never walk again, he agreed to an intrathecal catheter with bupivacaine, which provided excellent pain control. Bob was discharged home after a week in the acute care hospital and died a month later, surrounded by his family. Before his death, he was able to make amends with several estranged family members and was at peace in the end.

Although this was one of the more challenging cases that I ever managed, it also provided a rich opportunity for professional growth during the six months of collaboration. Lessons learned include the power of pure acceptance of a patient, just as he is, without trying to speed up his process of adjusting to illness; the power of listening carefully and without judgment, even if the patient's rationale for delay in treatment seems foolish; and the power of showing true kindness, warmth, and patience as a means to create a bridge to a "prickly" man's heart, which ultimately helped him die comfortably and at peace.

References

1. Smith AK, Thai JN, Bakitas MA, et al. The diverse landscape of palliative care clinics. *J Palliat Med.* 2013;16(6)661–668.

2. Meier DE, Beresford L. Outpatient clinics are a new frontier for palliative care. *J Palliat Med.* 2008;11(6):823–828.

3. Ferris FD, Bruera E, Cherny N, et al. Palliative cancer care a decade later: accomplishments, the need, next steps—from the American Society of Clinical Oncology. *J Clin Oncol.* 2009;27(18):3052–3058.

4 American Society of Clinical Oncology. ASCO Virtual Learning Collaborative. http://www.asco.org/quality-guidelines/asco-virtual-learning-collaborative. Accessed October 7, 2014.

5. Center to Advance Palliative Care. Improving Palliative Care—Outpatient (IPAL-OP). 2013. http://www.capc.org/ipal/ipal-op. Accessed October 7, 2014.

6. Malloy P, Virani R, Kelly K, Munévar C. Beyond bad news: communication skills of nurses in palliative care. *J Hospice Palliat Nurs.* 2010;12(3):166–174.

7. Quill TE, Abernethy AP. Generalist plus specialist palliative care: creating a more sustainable model. *N Engl J Med.* 2013;368(13):1173–1175.

8. von Gunten CF. Secondary and tertiary palliative care in US hospitals. *JAMA.* 2002;287(7):875–881.

9. Davies PS, Prince-Paul M. Palliative care in the outpatient cancer center: current trends. *J Hospice Palliat Nursing.* 2012;14(8):506–513.

10. Muir JC, Daly F, Davis MS, et al. Integrating palliative care into the outpatient, private practice oncology setting. *J Pain Symptom Manage.* 2010;40(1):126–135.

11. Rabow MW, Dibble SL, Pantilat SZ, McPhee SJ. The comprehensive care team: a controlled trial of outpatient palliative medicine consultation. *Archives of internal medicine.* 2004;164(1):83.

12. Murphy A, Siebert K, Owens D, Doorenbos A. Healthcare utilization by patients whose care is managed by a primary palliative care clinic. *J Hospice Palliat Nurs.* 2013;15(7):372–379.

13. Temel JS, Greer JA, Muzikansky A, et al. Early palliative care for patients with metastatic non–small-cell lung cancer. *N Engl J Med.* 2010;363(8):733–742.

14. Prince-Paul M, Burant CJ, Saltzman J, et al. The effects of integrating an advanced practice palliative care nurse in a community oncology center: a pilot study. *J Support Oncol.* 2010;8(1):21–27.

15. Bakitas M, Lyons KD, Hegel MT, et al. Effects of a palliative care intervention on clinical outcomes in patients with advanced cancer: the Project ENABLE II randomized controlled trial. *JAMA.* 2009;302(7):741–749.

16. Owens D, Eby K, Burson S, et al. Primary Palliative Care Clinic Pilot Project demonstrates benefits of a nurse practitioner directed clinic providing primary and palliative care. *J Am Acad Nurse Pract.* 2012;24(1):52–58.

17. Rabow MW, Smith AK, Braun JL, Weissman DE. Outpatient palliative care practices. *Arch Intern Med.* 2010;170(7):654–655.

18. National Comprehensive Cancer Network. *Clinical Practice Guideline in Oncology: Palliative Care.* 2013, http://www.nccn.org/professionals/physician_gls/f_guidelines.asp. Accessed October 27, 2014.

19. Weissman DE, Meier DE. Identifying patients in need of a palliative care assessment in the hospital setting: a consensus report from the center to advance palliative care. *J Palliat Med.* 2011;14(1):17–23.

20. Glare PA, Semple D, Stabler SM, Saltz LB. Palliative care in the outpatient oncology setting: evaluation of a practical set of referral criteria. *J Oncol Pract.* 2011;7(6):366–370.

21. Berger GN, O'Riordan DL, Kerr K, Pantilat SZ. Prevalence and characteristics of outpatient palliative care services in California. *Arch Intern Med.* 2011; 171(22):2057–2059.

22. Bookbinder M, Glajchen M, McHugh M, et al. Nurse practitioner-based models of specialist palliative care at home: sustainability and evaluation of feasibility. *J Pain Symptom Manage.* 2010;41(1):25–34.

23. Shah M, Quill T, Norton S, et al. "What bothers you the most?" Initial responses from patients receiving palliative care consultation. *Am J Hospice Palliat Med.* 2008;25(2):88–92.

24. Yoong J, Park ER, Greer JA, et al. Early palliative care in advanced lung cancer: a qualitative study. *JAMA.* 2013;173(4):283–290.

25. Von Roenn JH, Temel J. The integration of palliative care and oncology: the evidence. *Oncology.* 2011;25(13):1258–1266.

26. Jacobsen J, Jackson V, Dahlin C, et al. Components of early outpatient palliative care consultation in patients with metastatic nonsmall cell lung cancer. *J Palliat Med.* 2011;14(4):459–464.

27. Riechelmann RP, Krzyzanowska MK, O'Carroll A, Zimmermann C. Symptom and medication profiles among cancer patients attending a palliative care clinic. *Support Care Cancer.* 2007;15(12):1407–1412.

28. American Association of Colleges of Nursing. Peaceful death: recommended competencies and curricular guidelines for end of life nursing care. 2011. http://www.aacn.nche.edu/elnec/publications/peaceful-death. Accessed October 7, 2014.

29. Back AL, Arnold RM, Baile WF, et al. Approaching difficult communication tasks in oncology. *CA: Cancer J Clin.* 2005;55(3):164–177.

30. American Association of Colleges of Nursing. End of Life Nursing Education Consortium (ELNEC). 2013. http://www.aacn.nche.edu/elnec. Accessed October 7, 2014.

31. Schulman-Green D, McCorkle R, Cherlin E, et al. Nurses' communication of prognosis and implications for hospice referral: a study of nurses caring for terminally ill hospitalized patients. *Am J Crit Care.* 2005;14(1):64–70.

32. Fanslow-Brunjes C. Beyond pain: the search for hope in the patient's journey. *Asian Pacific J Cancer Prev.* 2010;11:63–66.

Chapter 6

Long-Term Care: Focus on Nursing Homes

Joan G. Carpenter and Mary Ersek

Quality end of life (EOL) care in nursing homes is important. In 2009, more than three million Americans lived in nursing homes.[1] More than half of these nursing home residents required extensive assistance or were completely dependent in bathing, dressing, toileting, and transferring. Despite the efforts to keep frail elders in the community, the nursing home population is expected to increase as the numbers of older persons in the United States and other developed countries grow larger. As more people live in nursing homes, for short or long periods, many will also die there. Although nursing homes were not established as sites for EOL care, increasingly they are becoming the place where many people die.

Challenges and Opportunities for Palliative Care Delivery in Nursing Homes

Despite the benefits, implementing palliative care philosophy and approaches to care in nursing homes are difficult. There are many barriers to delivering quality EOL care, although several characteristics facilitate the adoption of palliative care practices.[2]

Challenges to Palliative Care Delivery

Regulatory structures, reimbursement policies, workforce issues, and resident characteristics hamper efforts to expand the delivery of palliative care services in nursing homes. For example, regulations favor restorative rather than palliative care. There has been a remarkable growth in post-acute restorative nursing home care since 2001.[3] Efforts to administer palliative care sometimes are misinterpreted by facilities and regulators, leading to citations for poor care. For example, marked weight loss is an expected change toward the EOL and is rarely treated aggressively by palliative care and hospice teams. However, state surveyors who inspect nursing homes may interpret the loss as a sign of poor care.

Reimbursement also promotes more aggressive therapy. Generally, Medicaid and Medicare pay nursing homes a per diem amount for the care they provide rather than paying for the specific care provided. Specifics of care are instead accounted for in the facility's case mix index, a composite score reflecting the complexity of care delivered to residents. In facilities providing more medical interventions, therapy services, and assistance with activities of daily living, the case mix index and the reimbursement rates are higher. Therefore, facilities are financially incentivized to accept residents requiring "skilled" treatments. Intravenous therapies and tube feedings, for example, are reimbursed at a higher rate than alternative, less invasive therapies. These policies act as disincentives to nursing homes to provide palliative care services, even though these services may improve the overall quality of care and the residents' quality of life.[2]

In addition to regulatory and financial pressures, workforce issues are challenging. Nursing home staff tend to lack training in palliative care approaches and therefore have difficulties recognizing and implementing palliative treatments as appropriate. Unlicensed nursing assistants and licensed practical nurses (LPNs) or licensed vocational nurses (LVNs) provide the majority of direct care to residents, and their skills related to symptom assessment and treatment, communication, and decision-making are limited. Clinical decision-making is also somewhat fragmented because LPNs, LVNs, and nursing assistants often are minimally involved in developing care plans, even though they may know the residents best. As a result, symptoms may be poorly assessed and managed, families are dissatisfied, and residents are frequently subject to unnecessary and distressing medical interventions and hospitalizations.[2]

Another workforce issue is staff turnover, which is staggeringly high. In 2008, the annual turnover among nursing assistants was 53%, that of LPNs and registered nurses (RNs) was 43%, and that among directors of nursing was 18%. High turnover is associated with lack of care continuity and poorer care,[4] resulting in a workforce that is constantly changing, overwhelmed, and dissatisfied. It also requires offering educational programs on a continual basis to keep knowledge and skills current.[2]

Until recently, there was little empirical research investigating the direct correlation between staff turnover and the ability of nursing home staff to deliver high-quality EOL care. Using both quantitative and qualitative data, one research team was able to link high staff turnover to residents' poorer quality of dying. This inverse relationship was magnified with higher rates of turnover resulting in even poorer EOL care. Family members believed that the lack of staff contributed to worse quality of dying for their loved one.[5]

One strategy to address nursing assistant job satisfaction and improve EOL care is through continuing education programs. Researchers found statistically significant improvement in attitudes and knowledge about EOL care after a daylong education program.[6] Additional research, through surveys of hospice and palliative care nursing assistants, found that better compensation and improved relationships (e.g., communication, appreciation, respect) were perceived to improve job satisfaction.[7]

Finally, many residents have complex physical and psychosocial needs that are difficult to assess and manage because of cognitive impairment. Severe impairment interferes with residents' ability to provide reliable self-report, thereby hindering pain and symptom assessment and management. When pain and other symptoms are identified, multiple comorbidities and polypharmacy further complicate effective treatment.

Facilitators to Providing Palliative Care

Although there are hindrances, several nursing home characteristics facilitate palliative care delivery. These factors include relatively long stays and daily interaction between direct care staff and residents, the existing team approach to care, family meetings, and use of the Minimum Data Set (MDS).[2]

Daily interaction between staff and residents, who are familiar with each other, establishes a rich context for developing relationships congruent with palliative care philosophy. Nursing assistants who care for residents from day-to-day have greater knowledge of resident routines, likes and dislikes, and needs. Residents are often more comfortable and accustomed to caregivers who know them well. Frequently, nursing home staff describe themselves as part of the resident's family.[8] These close relationships can improve mutual understanding of residents' goals of care, values, and preferences and result in better symptom management.

The existing interdisciplinary team (IDT)—RNs, LPNs, nursing assistants, social worker, rehabilitation specialists, dietitian, and wound care specialists—supports the palliative care philosophy. The best approach to care for older adults with life-limiting illness is through multiple professionals working together for a common purpose—to meet a resident's goal of care. Unmet psychosocial support and spiritual needs can be addressed in this forum by social workers and pastoral care staff.

Nursing homes are required to hold regular meetings with residents and/or their family members to discuss the comprehensive physical, emotional, mental, and social care plan for each resident. The plan focuses on objectives that maintain the resident's highest level of function. Ideally, at the point when the highest level of function is not maintained, the nursing home staff, resident, and/or family should discuss revising goals of care.

The MDS is a mandated assessment tool for Medicare and Medicaid beneficiaries in nursing homes. The goal of this tool is to create a comprehensive evaluation and to identify opportunities to improve functional status. MDS 3.0 is a revised tool that builds on previous versions, using resident input or "voice" in assessments. The tool is completed by an RN at specified intervals using medical records, staff input, and observation, in combination with a resident interview. The resident interview consists of discussions of preferences for routines and activities, including goals of care, and questions about pain, mood, and cognition.[9] The MDS can be used to identify residents with life-limiting illness who have unmet symptom management and psychospiritual support needs. These residents are candidates for palliative care. The crucial next step after identifying palliative care needs is the delivery of care that matches the resident's goals of treatment.

Models to Deliver Palliative Care in Nursing Homes

There is a shortage of evidence-based research in palliative care delivery models in nursing homes. In contrast, there is a great deal of evidence about the effectiveness of palliative care teams in acute care settings. Palliative care teams have been shown to reduce healthcare costs by avoiding unwanted or undesired treatments and increase satisfaction, using person-centered patient care.[10-13] Meier and Beresford[14] asserted that the benefits of palliative care can also be achieved in nursing homes.

The Center to Advance Palliative Care (CAPC) compiled anecdotal evidence for successful palliative care delivery models in nursing homes and reported their findings in 2008.[15] These programs can be categorized into three major approaches: hospice–nursing home partnerships, external palliative care consultation teams, and in-house teams and specialized palliative care units.[2]

Hospice Care in Nursing Homes

Hospice care is the most common and well-established program for delivering palliative care in U.S. nursing homes. The Medicare Hospice Benefit (MHB) was extended to nursing homes in 1989, and by 2004, 78% of nursing homes reported a contract with a hospice agency.[16] Hospice, with the MHB, is the traditional program for delivering EOL care to individuals with terminal illness. Nursing home residents must meet hospice admission criteria: a life expectancy of six months or less should the terminal illness run its usual course and a decision not to pursue aggressive "curative" treatments.

In nursing homes, the MHB pays the hospice agency to oversee the plan of care and provide all medical supplies and medications related to the terminal condition. Medicare pays the hospice agency for care related to the terminal illness. The facility continues to deliver 24-hour nursing care for the resident. The MHB does not provide the resident's payment for room and board—the most expensive component of nursing home care. Only rarely can residents access the Medicare skilled nursing facility (SNF) care benefit and MHB at the same time (e.g., unrelated diagnoses for each benefit). Some suggest that this barrier incentivizes families to choose the benefit with greater financial support.[17,18]

Hospice is often described as an "extra layer of support" for residents. The use of hospice in nursing homes is associated with improved symptom management, reduced hospitalizations, and increased satisfaction with care. Research comparing EOL care for residents with and without hospice demonstrates that hospice care is associated with better psychosocial support, bereavement care, and pain management.[19,20] Facility leadership reported improved ability to manage pain and symptoms, address psychosocial needs, and provide bereavement support when a formal program, such as hospice, is integrated into the facility culture.[21]

The challenge for hospice agencies, facilities, and providers is that a majority of nursing home residents have a life-limiting illness with an uncertain trajectory, making it difficult to decide when the illness is "terminal" according to existing guidelines. Persons with dementia and neurologic conditions experience a long, slow disease progression, with eventual complete dependence on others for daily living. Those with chronic respiratory and cardiac illness have frequent exacerbations that require acute care and result in diminished capacity during recovery. As a result, residents live with frailty and are susceptible to aggressive treatments that may not align with their values and goals of care.

There are other barriers to enrolling residents in hospice. Nursing home administrators and staff may believe that bringing hospice services into the facility indicates that their own care is inadequate.[22] Furthermore, poor communication and lack of collegial relationships can compromise care and engender discord between nursing home and hospice staff. Additionally, there are financial disincentives for nursing homes to transfer residents who were admitted under the Medicare SNF benefit to the MHB because the reimbursement is much lower for the MHB.[23]

External Consultation Teams

External palliative care consultation teams provide specialized services in nursing homes and make recommendations for the resident's care. Consultation teams can be an extension of existing hospital-based teams, outpatient teams, or independent practitioners. Depending on the team and resources, consultations may focus on symptom management, advance care planning, or assisting with prognostication and/or hospice entry. Need for a consult is typically identified by staff or leadership, then formally requested by the primary care provider. The consultant bills under Medicare Part B, and thus, the costs for these services are not incurred by the nursing home.

The outcome of consultation is dependent on several factors. First, the consulting clinician needs to understand the nursing home environment and have knowledge of interventions that can and cannot be carried out. For example, some palliative care medications are not on nursing home formularies. In addition, the ability to administer and titrate intravenous opioids may be limited. Second, implementing recommendations depends on the primary care provider's willingness to accept and implement palliative care recommendations.[15] Third, nursing homes are unique settings, and few are exactly the same. Depending on the underlying culture, facility staff may not be comfortable implementing EOL care.[2]

Integrated Palliative Care

Some nursing facilities report the presence of an internal palliative care team, services, or unit. In 2004, 27% of nursing home respondents reported having a special program and staff for hospice, palliative care, and/or EOL care.[16] Incorporating palliative care into daily routines requires a commitment to person-centered care and improving EOL care.[17] Benefits of this model have been reported for residents and staff alike, including a reduction in resident medication use and staff empowerment.[23,24] Culture change and integrated palliative care share several characteristics, including person-centered care and practices that maximize choice (i.e., autonomy) and individualized care.

A major hindrance to developing internal nursing home palliative care services is the lack of resources. The need to train staff and the extra time required to deliver high-quality palliative care are additional barriers. Also, there are no financial incentives to provide high-quality palliative care because the highest reimbursement rates are for post-acute, skilled care.[2]

Specific Strategies for Enhancing Palliative Care

Some nursing homes incorporate specific palliative care approaches in addition to, or instead of, comprehensive models. These targeted areas often are pain management, advance care planning, and interventions to decrease hospitalizations.

Pain and other symptoms are common in nursing home residents. Evidence from several studies show that pain occurs in 40% to 86% of residents[25]: dyspnea in 11% to 75%,[25,26] feeding problems in 28% to 70%,[25,26] delirium in 29% to 47%,[25,26] incontinence in 59%,[25] and noisy breathing in 39% to 59%.[25] Several studies provide evidence that these symptoms often are inadequately managed.[26,27]

Several intervention trials to improve pain management have been conducted. These studies used a variety of approaches, including quality improvement, pain management algorithms, specialized pain teams, and staff education.[27] The effectiveness of these approaches has been mixed. Moreover, there are no high-quality trials of interventions aimed at non-pain symptoms. Despite the lack of empirical evidence on effective ways to change pain and symptom management practices, many excellent resources are available to promote quality symptom assesment and management in nursing homes (Table 6.1.)

Advance Care Planning

The number of nursing home residents with advance directives increased dramatically over the past 15 years. Jones and colleagues[28] reported that 65% of nursing home residents had an advance directive in 2004 (the most recent year for which there are national data). Advance directives, in the form of a living will and durable power of attorney for healthcare, are completed by residents while they have decision-making capacity. When a resident lacks medical decision-making capacity, a resident's family member (acting as an appointed healthcare agent or surrogate decision-maker) will ideally use the advance directive to guide decisions on medical treatments and EOL care. Most advance directives for older nursing home residents reflect preferences for less aggressive EOL care.[28]

Table 6.1 Palliative Care Resources for Nursing Home Nursing Staff and Other Providers

Resource	Description
End of Life Nursing Education Consortium (ELNEC) geriatric curriculum	Comprehensive training for nurses and nursing assistants, as well as social workers, chaplains, and others working in nursing homes Also useful for hospice staff who serve nursing homes Website: http://www.aacn.nche.edu/elnec
Advancing Excellence in America's Nursing Homes	Initiative of the Advancing Excellence in Long Term Care Collaborative; goal of the campaign is to ensure quality of care and quality of life for nursing home residents. Website contains resources on palliative care topics such as advance care planning and pain assessment and management, organized within a quality improvement framework. Website https://www.nhqualitycampaign.org/
Core Curriculum for the Long-Term Care Nurse	Comprehensive curriculum in detailed outline, book format Organized by the National Consensus Project Domains Website: www.nationalconsensusproject.org Available from the Hospice and Palliative Nurses Association: http://hpna.org/Item_Details.aspx?ItemNo= 978-1-934654-30-9
Nursing Education Computerized Education Program	Comprehensive curriculum for nursing assistants working in any setting CD contains text, audio clips, video clips, a pop-up glossary, quizzes, and printable pdf files Available from the Hospice and Palliative Nurses Association: http://hpna.org/Item_Details. aspx?ItemNo=NACDROM
Palliative Care in the Long Term Care Setting	Developed for medical directors and primary care providers in nursing homes Contains a variety of resources to improve palliative and end of life care through leadership, education, best practice guidelines, and quality assurance Available from the American Medical Directors Association: http://amda.com/resources/ltcis.cfm#LTCPC1
Geriatric Pain website	Website containing evidence-based materials to guide nurses and other nursing home staff in assessing and managing residents' pain, including residents with dementia Website: http://www.geriatricpain.org/Pages/home.aspx
Palliative Care for Advanced Dementia Teaching Unit	Developed by the Beatitudes Campus Dementia and Aging Research Department and Hospice of the Valley in Phoenix, AZ, this interdisciplinary program specifically targets the knowledge and skills needed to provide person-centered, comfort care to persons with dementia and their families. Website: http://www.beatitudescampus.org/ health-services/memory-support/
ConsultGeriRN	Website with articles and videos relevant to the care of older adults, including pain assessment in nonverbal persons and avoiding restraint use Website: http://consultgerirn.org/resources

Although preferences about resuscitation are commonly documented, decisions about other interventions, such as artificial nutrition and hydration, hospitalization, antibiotics, and comfort measures, are not.[29] The use of the Physician Orders for Life-Sustaining Treatment (POLST) is one effective way of encouraging discussion about, and documentation of, residents' and families' decisions about specific therapeutic approaches.[30] Moreover, the POLST paradigm increases concordance between residents' or families' preferences and care received. Other effective strategies are the use of social workers, with specialized training in advance directives and facilitating goals of care discussions, and implementation of the "Let Me Decide" advance directive program.[31]

End of Life Transitions

Several studies have documented that many nursing home residents are hospitalized in the final weeks of life[32,33] and receive burdensome treatments with little benefit, including tube feeding[34] and post-acute, rehabilitative care.[17,18]

To address this problem, Ouslander and colleagues[35] used a pre-post intervention design to examine the effectiveness of several treatment algorithms and other tools designed to reduce hospitalizations. Findings from this quality improvement program indicated that these tools can decrease hospitalization rates and healthcare costs. Packaged into a program, the Interventions to Reduce Acute Care Transfers (INTERACT) tools[36] are now being examined in several ongoing nursing home demonstration projects funded by the Center for Medicare and Medicaid Innovations (CMMI) (http://innovation.cms.gov/initiatives/rahnfr/index.html).

Another promising approach to decreasing hospitalizations and promoting comfort was tested in a cluster randomized controlled trial conducted by Loeb and colleagues.[37] The study compared the effects of a nursing home–based clinical pathway for pneumonia treatment, with usual care, on hospitalizations, length of hospital stay, mortality, health-related quality of life, functional status, and cost. Results showed that the pneumonia clinical pathway was associated with significantly fewer hospitalizations, shorter lengths of hospital stay, and lower costs compared with usual care.

Resources for Enhancing Palliative Care in Nursing Homes

Over the past several years, many professional and industry groups have developed curricula, websites, and other palliative care resources for nursing homes. Many of these resources are training materials which have been shown to increase nursing home staffs' knowledge and skills.[38] Table 6.1 presents information about several of these resources.

References

1. Center for Medicare and Medicaid Services. Nursing Home Data Compendium. 8th ed. 2010. http://www.cms.gov/Medicare/Provider-Enrollment-and-Certification/CertificationandComplianc/downloads/nursinghomedatacompendium_508.pdf. Accessed October 27, 2014.

2. Sefcik J, Rao A, Ersek M. What models exist for delivering palliative care and hospice in nursing homes? In: Goldstein N, Morrison R, eds. *Evidence-Based Practice of Palliative Medicine*. Philadelphia: Elsevier; 2013:450–457.

3. Tyler DA, Feng Z, Leland NE, et al. Trends in postacute care and staffing in US nursing homes, 2001-2010. *J Am Med Dir Assoc*. 2013;14(11):817–820.

4. Harrington C, Carrillo H, Blank B. Nursing facilities, staffing, residents and facility deficiencies, 2001 through 2007. http://ualr.edu/seniorjustice/uploads/2008/12/Nursing%20Home%20Facilities,%20Staffing,%20Residents,%20and%20Facility%20Deficiencies%202001%20Through%20 2007.pdf. Accessed October 8, 2014.

5. Tilden V, Thompson S, Gajewski B, Bott M. End of life care in nursing homes: the high cost of staff turnover. *Nurs Econ*. 2012;30(3):163–166.

6. Wholihan D, Anderson R. empowering nursing assistants to improve end of life care. *J Hosp Palliat Nurs*. 2013;15(1):24–32.

7. Head BA, Washington KT, Myers J. Job satisfaction, intent to stay, and recommended job improvements: the palliative nursing assistant speaks. *J Palliat Med*. 2013;16(11):1356–1361.

8. Ersek M, Sefcik, J., Stevenson, D. Palliative care in nursing homes. In: Kelley AM, DE, ed. *Meeting the Needs of Older Adults with Serious Illness: Clinical, Public Health, and Policy Perspectives*. New York: Springer; 2014:73–90.

9. Saliba D, Buchanan J. *Development and Validation of a Revised Nursing Home Assessment Tool: MDS 3.0*. Santa Monica: RAND Health; 2008.

10. Smith TJ, Cassel JB. Cost and non-clinical outcomes of palliative care. *J Pain Sympt Manage*. 2009;38(1):32–44.

11. Morrison RS, Penrod J, Cassel B, et al. Cost savings associated with US hospital palliative care consultation programs. *Arch Intern Med*. 2008;168(6):1783–1790.

12. Morrison RS, Dietrich J, Ladwig S, et al. Palliative care consultation teams cut hospital costs for medicaid beneficiaries. *Health Affairs*. 2011;30(3): 454–463.

13. Cassel JB, Webb-Wright J, Holmes J, et al. Clinical and financial impact of a palliative care program at a small rural hospital. *J Palliat Med*. 2010;13(11):1339–1343.

14. Meier DE, Beresford L. Palliative care in long-term care: how can hospital teams interface? *J Palliat Med*. 2010;13(2):111–115.

15. Center to Advance Palliative Care. *Improving Palliative Care in Nursing Homes*. New York, NY: Center to Advance Palliative Care; 2008.

16. Miller SC, Han B. End of life care in U.S. nursing homes: nursing nomes with special programs and trained staff for hospice or palliative/end of life care. *J Palliat Med*. 2008;11(6):866–877.

17. Aragon K, Covinsky K, Miao Y, et al. Use of the Medicare posthospitalization skilled nursing benefit in the last 6 months of life. *Arch Intern Med*. 2012; 172(20):1573–1579.

18. Miller SC, Lima JC, Mitchell SL. Influence of hospice on nursing home residents with advanced dementia who received Medicare-skilled nursing facility care near the end of life. *J Am Geriatr Soc.* 2012;60(11):2035–2041.

19. Miller SC, Lima JC, Looze J, Mitchell SL. Dying in U.S. nursing homes with advanced dementia: how does healthcare use differ for residents with, versus without, end of life Medicare skilled nursing facility care? *J Palliat Med.* 2012;15(1):43–50.

20. Huskamp H, Kaufmann C, Stevenson D. The intersection of long-term care and end of life care. *Med Care Res Rev.* 2012;69(1):45–57.

21. Rice KN, Coleman EA, Fish R, et al. Factors influencing models of end of life care in nursing homes: Results of a survey of nursing home administrators. *J Palliat Med.* 2004;7(5):668–675.

22. Stevenson DG, Bramson JS. Hospice care in the nursing home setting: a review of the literature. *J Pain Symptom Manage.* 2009;38(3):440–451.

23. Suhrie EM, Hanlon JT, Jaffe EJ, et al. Impact of a geriatric nursing home palliative care service on unnecessary medication prescribing. *Am J Geriatr Pharmacother.* 2009;7(1):20–25.

24. Stone R, Harahan MF. Improving the long-term care workforce serving older adults. *Health Affairs.* 2010;29(1):109–115.

25. Brandt HE, Deliens L, Ooms ME, et al. Symptoms, signs, problems, and diseases of terminally ill nursing home patients: a nationwide observational study in the Netherlands. *Arch Intern Med.* 2005;165(3):314–320.

26. Hanson LC, Eckert JK, Dobbs D, et al. Symptom experience of dying long-term care residents. *J Am Geriatr Soc.* 2008;56:91–98.

27. Ersek M, Carpenter JG. Research priorities for geriatric palliative care in long-term care settings with a focus on nursing homes. *J Palliat Med.* 2013;16(10):1180–1187.

28. Jones A, Moss A, Harris-Kojetin L. *Use of Advance Directives in Long-term Care Populations.* NCHS Data Brief, No. 54. Hyattsville, MD: National Center for Health Statistics; 2011.

29. Levy CR, Fish R, Kramer A. Do-not-resuscitate and do-not-hospitalize directives of persons admitted to skilled nursing facilities under the Medicare benefit. *J Am Geriatr Soc.* 2005;53(12):2060–2068.

30. Hickman SE, Nelson CA, Perrin NA, et al. A comparison of methods to communicate treatment preferences in nursing facilities: traditional practices versus the physician orders for life-sustaining treatment program. *J Am Geriatr Soc.* 2010;58(7):1241–1248.

31. Molloy DW, Guyatt GH, Russo R, et al. Systematic implementation of an advance directive program in nursing homes: a randomized controlled trial. *JAMA.* 2000;283(11):1437–1444.

32. Gozalo P, Teno JM, Mitchell SL, et al. End of life transitions among nursing home residents with cognitive issues. *N Engl J Med.* 2011;365(13):1212–1221.

33. Ouslander JG, Lamb G, Perloe M, et al. Potentially avoidable hospitalizations of nursing home residents: frequency, causes, and costs. *J Am Geriatr Soc.* 2010;58(4):627–635. *See editorial comments by Drs. Jean F. Wyman and William R. Hazzard, pp. 760–761.*

34. Teno JM, Mitchell SL, Gozalo PL, et al. Hospital characteristics associated with feeding tube placement in nursing home residents with advanced cognitive impairment. *JAMA.* 2010;303(6):544–550.

35. Ouslander JG, Lamb G, Tappen R, et al. Interventions to reduce hospitalizations from nursing homes: evaluation of the INTERACT II collaborative quality improvement project. *J Am Geriatr Soc*. 2011;59(4):745–753.

36. Interventions to Reduce Acute Care Transfers: INTERACT. 2011. http://interact2.net/index.aspx. Accessed October 8, 2014.

37. Loeb M, Carusone SC, Goeree R, et al. Effect of a clinical pathway to reduce hospitalizations in nursing home residents with pneumonia: a randomized controlled trial. *JAMA*. 2006;295(21):2503–2510.

38. Ersek M, Grant MM, Kraybill BM. Enhancing end of life care in nursing homes: Palliative Care Educational Resource Team (PERT) program. *J Palliat Med*. 2005;8(3):556–566.

Chapter 7

Clinical Interventions, Economic Impact, and Palliative Care

Patrick J. Coyne, Thomas J. Smith, and Laurie J. Lyckholm

Healthcare spending and healthcare quality are major challenges in the United States, with healthcare spending reaching nearly $8,000 per person per year, twice that of most other countries with similar health outcomes. In the United States, health expenditures neared $2.6 trillion in 2010, more than ten times the $256 billion spent in 1980.[1] The growth rate in recent years has slowed compared with the late 1990s and early 2000s, but in the coming years, it is still expected to grow faster than national income.[2] Drug costs and rising hospital expenses fuel much of this spending.[1-7]

Employer-sponsored health coverage premiums have increased by up to 97%, placing increased cost burdens on both employers and workers.[3] Medicare covers elderly people and people with disabilities, and Medicaid provides coverage to low-income individuals and families. Enrollment has increased with the aging of the baby boomers, which is presenting ongoing economic challenges.[1,4] Twenty percent of Medicare beneficiaries have five or more chronic illnesses and consume 60% of the Medicare spending.[5] This has had a considerable impact on our government's spending, straining federal and state budgets. Health spending accounted for 17.9% of the nation's gross domestic product (GDP) in 2010.[5] Although the United States spends more on healthcare than other industrialized nations, those countries provide health insurance to all their citizens. A 2013 study found that about 25% of all senior citizens who declare bankruptcy do so because of medical expenses.[8] About 84 million Americans are uninsured or underinsured, three million more than when the 2010 health law was signed, and 20 million more than in 2003.[9] As of January 2011, *there are more than eight million uninsured children in the United States.*[10] Increasing healthcare costs correlate to health insurance coverage reductions[3].

We spend too much money on healthcare near the end of life, the quality is often poor, and it not what most people want. About one-fourth of all Medicare dollars are spent in the last year of life, and 40% of that is spent in the last *month* of life—at least 8% of all Medicare dollars.[11] Teno and colleagues[12] have shown actual *increases* in intensive care unit

(ICU) use, in the last 30 days of life, for Medicare-age people who die. Twenty-nine percent use the ICU in the last month of life, and only 42% of patients with a terminal illness use hospice at any time during their illness. As patients transition out of intensive care, 14% have a change of healthcare setting in the last three days of life. This may involve transfer from hospital to home or hospital to inpatient hospice. The last few days of life are probably the worst time to disrupt families and to expect them to form new and trusting relationships. In addition, Kelley and colleagues[13] reported that even with Medicare coverage, elderly households face considerable financial risk from out-of-pocket healthcare expenses at the end of life.

There are, however, substantial concerns about the quality of palliative care in our current healthcare system. The Study to Understand Prognoses and Preferences for Outcomes and Risks of Treatments (SUPPORT) showed that half of all dying patients had unnecessary pain and suffering in their final days of life, while in the hospital.[14] Pooled data from 52 articles reveals that pain was prevalent in cancer patients: 64% in patients with metastatic or advanced-stage disease, 59% in patients on anticancer treatment, and 33% in patients after curative treatment. In the reviewed articles, more than one-third of the patients with pain graded their pain as moderate or severe. Nearly one of two patients with cancer pain is undertreated.[15] The percentage is high but consists of a large variability of undertreatment across studies and settings. Despite 20 years of interventions, 33% of current cancer patients have inadequate analgesics prescribed, with rates even higher in minority patients.[16,17]

Although it is not a zero-sum situation, there is good evidence that the more that is spent on high-technology care for elderly people, the fewer funds are available for preventive services or treatment of chronic disease conditions for the same population.[16] The drain on healthcare–directed funds is likely to increase because of heightened demands from an educated, elderly population, more elderly long-term survivors, new and expensive technologies, new diseases, and demands for cost cutting. Many U.S. lawmakers, including conservative physician and ex-Senator Dr. William Frist, have called on us to confront our mortality and plan for a "good death" as part of personal responsibility.[18]

The Patient Protection and Affordable Care Act (Public Law 111-148) was signed into law in the United States by President Barack Obama on March 23, 2010. Along with the Health Care and Education Reconciliation Act of 2010 (passed March 25, 2010), the Act is a product of the healthcare reform agenda of the Democratic 111th Congress and the Obama administration. The goal of the Act is to ensure that all Americans have access to affordable healthcare and to create the transformation within the healthcare system to control cost. When fully paid for, the Congressional Budget Office (CBO) has determined that it will provide coverage for more than 94% of Americans. The law includes a large number of health-related provisions to take effect over the next four years, including expanding Medicaid's role.

Where Does Palliative Care Fit into the Economic Equation?

The present, average life expectancy is 78 years. Many individuals will develop chronic illnesses such as heart failure, emphysema, stroke, dementia, and cancer. They will live with these conditions for many years before they die.[6] In the adult population, degenerative diseases replaced communicable diseases as leading causes of death in the United States and most economically advanced countries. The 10 leading causes of death (in order of prevalence) accounted for 80% of all deaths in the United States in 2008.[19] The majority of these individuals will benefit from palliative care at some point in their disease trajectory. As shown later in this chapter, palliative care is one of the rare aspects of medicine that improves the patient experience, maintains or improves survival, improves the quality of care (especially concerning end of life care hospitalizations), and saves money.[20]

Ethics of Adding Economic Outcomes for the Provision of Palliative Care

Although quality care is the primary goal of hospice and palliative medicine, cost control is an important consideration. Nursing and medicine aspire to promote health and provide comfort and relief of suffering in a just manner. Cost control through evidence-based disease management, or "critical paths," may actually promote these goals by making more and/or better care available.

Cost control must be differentiated from profit motivation and entrepreneurship, which have not traditionally been considered the goals of medicine. These activities, in the context of healthcare, are unethical in that they may make medical care more expensive and difficult to access, especially for those who are socially disadvantaged. They may also create further conflicts of interest in already precarious fiduciary relationships between clinicians and their patients. A code of ethics that covers all professionals, rather than medicine alone, might be useful.[21-26] Nursing has its own code of ethics, as do other disciplines.

If palliative care can be improved and/or made less costly without sacrificing quality, it should be done in the service of promoting the values of beneficence, compassion, and respect for autonomy. Palliative care has emerged as a national movement, with the advent of several important initiatives (e.g., Oncology Nursing Society; Hospice and Palliative Nurses Association; Education for Physicians on End of Life Care; and the End of Life Nursing Education Consortium). Other well-established national resource educational programs include the National Palliative Care Resource Center; City of Hope, CA; the Center to Improve Care of the Dying at George Washington University, Washington, DC; and the Center to Advance Palliative Care at Mount Sinai Hospital in New York, NY. In addition, palliative care programs continue to develop all over the world. In the United States, more than 80% of large hospitals have palliative care programs.[27]

Some have argued that budgets should not be balanced with penalty to one group, such as elderly people or those on Medicare.[23] Many healthcare goods are rationed justly (benefit vs. risk) according to age, such as transplantation, coronary bypass, and hemodialysis. This rationing is based on the theory of equality of opportunity, according to the ability to benefit from such procedures.[24] Palliative care is different, however, in that age does not determine whether a person stands to benefit. In this circumstance, the ethic of distributive justice supports the concept that medical and social needs dictate who stands to benefit most from palliative care. Daniels[25] reported that "it does not seem reasonable to postulate that the medical needs of the elderly terminally ill are any less than those of younger patients, and indeed, they may be greater because of multiple additional pathologies associated with aging." Sidgwick's[26] argument that each moment of life is equally valuable, no matter when it occurs, is most poignant in the instance of palliative care. This would also apply to extending palliative care to neonates expected to live only a short time after birth. For adults, the most explicitly described guidance is from the United Kingdom's National Institute for Clinical Excellence (NICE), which gives guidance on what treatments the National Health Service should fund, given a fixed budget. NICE allows for special consideration if the expected patient survival is short, and may waive the usual three-month survival benefit if the treatment gives substantial palliative benefit at a reasonable cost.[28]

Patients may view benefit and toxicity in ways very different from their healthcare providers and from those who are well. Studies show that many dying cancer patients would undergo almost any treatment toxicity for a 1% chance of short-term survival, whereas their doctors and nurses would not; and these decisions did not change after patients experienced the toxicity of treatment.[29,30] If the patient wants to try a therapy with minimal chance of benefit, we should not assume that the oncologist or cardiologist has not adequately explained the options, risks, and benefits—the patient may just have a different perspective.

What Is the Right Amount to Spend on Healthcare?

How much to spend on healthcare cannot be determined without knowing the economic and cultural particulars of a country or even a health system. Blanket statements about a percentage of the GNP may be misleading, if a comparison country spends a higher percentage on social safety net programs, but less on direct medical care costs. Comments about healthcare spending as a percentage of the GNP may also reflect opinions about alternative uses—for example, "We should stop spending money on defense and spend it on healthcare." In the United States, the amount spent on education has declined from 6% to 5% of the GNP, whereas the amount spent on healthcare (especially for elderly people) has risen from 6% to about 18%, compared with the 9.5% average of 33 other developed countries.[31] Clearly, in all countries, the entire system of healthcare needs to be explored and policies designed to ensure that palliative care is a component of the overall healthcare system. A common threshold is the World Health Organization (WHO) recommendation of three times per-capita GNP per quality-adjusted life year, or how much we should spend to save a year of life; in the United States, that would be about $140,100 in 2008 U.S. dollars.

Should There Be Special Economic or Policy Considerations for Palliative Care?

We believe that, in general, there should be no special considerations for palliative care. Most healthcare policy analysts and economists would argue that all care should be evaluated equally. For example, a therapy that gains one week of life for 52 patients should be valued as much as a therapy of equivalent cost that gains 52 weeks of life for 1 patient.[32] Some health economists have argued that time given to those who are most at-risk should be valued more (e.g., time added in the last six months of life should be given triple value).[32] The analogy was made to food and hunger: a sandwich given to a starving person would be of more intrinsic value than one given to a person who already had many sandwiches. Such discussions, although interesting, are outside the scope of this chapter and will remain unresolved.

The WHO advocates a more equal distribution of resources in developed countries and an even greater support of palliative care in developing countries, where most of the population will experience advanced disease, rather than cure or long-term survival.

One approach to funding treatments has been based on cost-effectiveness ratios. For example, Laupacis and colleagues[33] in Canada proposed explicit funding criteria: (1) treatments that are more effective and less expensive should be adopted; (2) treatments with cost-effectiveness ratios of less than C$20,000 per additional life year (LY) gained should be accepted, with the recognition that they cost additional resources; (3) treatments with cost-effectiveness ratios of $20,000 to C$100,000/LY should be examined on a case-by-case basis with caution; and (4) treatments with cost-effectiveness ratios of greater than C$100,000/LY should be rejected. These criteria are valid in a system where all resources are shared equally, such as the Veterans Administration with a fixed budget, but it is not clear how they apply to other healthcare systems, in which resources may not be shared. Alternatively, patients might be allowed to purchase additional insurance for expensive treatments or pay for them out of pocket. In the United States, there has been no accepted answer, but most authorities have agreed on an implicitly defined benchmark of $35,000 to $50,000/LY saved, updated to $180,000 to $240,000 in current dollars.

Palliative care rarely costs more and usually saves money for better care. As an example, in England, home-based palliative care allowed patients to avoid emergency department visits, while promoting appropriate care with apparent cost savings of 40%.[34] A specially designed palliative care program for multiple sclerosis patients not only improved symptoms, but saved the National Health Service more than $2,700 in a 12-week trial period, from reduced hospitalizations.[35]

What Are Important Economic Outcomes?

Economic and clinical outcomes are closely related. Cost should always be considered along with clinical benefit. However, making decisions is not easy. The economic data necessary to make decisions about treatment may be collected in much the same way as clinical information and within standard formats for collection and analysis. Some standard definitions are listed in Table 7.1.

Table 7.1 Standard Definitions for Economic Outcome Analysis		
Term	**Definition**	**Comment**
Resource utilization	Number of units used (e.g., nine hospital days)	Best collected prospectively, using a combination of clinical research forms, hospital bills, and patient diaries for outpatient or off-site events
Charge	What is billed to the patient	May be fair representation of the cost of service
Cost	What it costs society to provide the service	This is different from the charge because many services cost more or less than what is billed
Direct medical cost	Costs of standard medical interventions	Usual "cost drivers" include hospital days, professional fees, diagnostic tests, pharmacy fees, other (e.g., blood products, operating room, emergency services).
Direct nonmedical cost	Costs of medical interventions not usually captured but directly caused	Includes transportation, time lost from work, caregiver costs, etc. Most are not covered by insurance and may be out-of-pocket costs.
Perspective	The viewpoint of the analysis	Should be explicitly stated. Most analyses are done from the perspective of society (valuing this intervention vs. other uses of the same money) or a healthcare system (valuing this intervention against other local healthcare needs). The perspective of the individual patient or provider may give less attention to the needs of others.[36]
Discounting	Adjusts value of intervention for future benefit to present-time amount	Health effects and costs should normally be discounted at 3% per year. Health benefits in the present are worth more than those in the future.

Source: Smith TJ. Which hat do I wear? *JAMA.* 1993;270:1657-1659. Copyright © 1993, American Medical Association. All rights reserved.

It is important to organize data in a way that balances clinical and cost information side-by-side. As shown in Table 7.2, cost effectiveness is the amount of money someone must pay to gain additional months or years of life. The usual benchmark is "life years gained," or LYs. If the amount of time is adjusted for quality, for instance, a year with advanced metastatic disease is only valued at 50%, or 6 months, then quality-adjusted life years (QALYs) are used.

Some countries, such as Canada, the United Kingdom, Australia, Germany, and France, use these metrics to inform decisions on what can be afforded. Oregon used cost effectiveness to inform their list of covered services under Medicaid, ultimately incorporating other values into the equation. The decision-making process is never easy because it always means withholding some desired care. However, all health systems make such decisions now, such as a Pharmacy and Therapeutics Committee; the life-years method just makes the decision-making transparent. We predict a growing emphasis on explicit sharing of effectiveness and cost

Table 7.2 Ways to Balance Clinical Evaluation and Cost Studies	
Type of Study	**Advantages and Disadvantages[35]**
Clinical outcomes only	Ignore costs. Easy to choose among clearly superior therapies such as cisplatin for testicular cancer that do not cost much; harder among all others that give lesser benefits at high costs.
Cost only (e.g., cost of treating febrile neutropenia)	Ignores clinical outcomes. Does not help choose among clinical strategies.
Costs and clinical outcomes together	
Cost minimization	Assumes that two strategies are equal; lowest cost strategy is preferred. If generic paclitaxel is as good as expensive ixabepilone in breast cancer, choose the $60 one, not the $6000 one.
Cost-effectiveness	Compares two strategies; assigns dollar amount per additional year of life (life year [LY]) saved by strategy. Example: at present, CSFs have not improved survival, so cost must be lower for therapy to be cost-effective.
Cost utility	Compares two strategies; assigns dollar amount per additional LY saved by strategy, then estimates the quality of that benefit in cost per quality adjusted LY. No data show significant improvement in quality of life or utilities in patients who have received CSFs, so they are unlikely to have major impact.
Cost benefit	Compares two strategies but converts the clinical benefits to money (e.g., a year of life is worth $100,000). This is possible but is rarely done because of difficulty in assigning monetary value to benefit; it requires assigning a monetary value to human life. For instance, should a bus driver's life be valued less than a physicist's life, or vice versa?

information with patients as the cost of treatments goes up in order to help them decide whether a treatment is "worth it."

Models of Care and Cost that Maintain Quality and Lower Cost

Coordinated care may be one of the most economically successful disease-management strategies. For instance, a large U.S. practice created evidence-based clinical pathways with an emphasis on (1) use of generic drugs, (2) restricting treatments to those based on solid evidence, (3) incorporating increased use of advance directives, and (4) earlier hospice referral. As a result, patient survival is the same or even better with less fourth- and fifth-line chemotherapy, hospice use is increased, and cost is reduced by one-third.

Recent randomized studies show that a modified palliative care presence (with lower costs than full hospice care per diem charges) and control over the clinical care of the patient are associated with fewer hospitalizations, fewer ICU hospital days, and lower costs. Brumley and colleagues[36] studied patients in the Kaiser Permanente health maintenance organization: 161 in the Palliative Care Program and 139 in the comparison group. Palliative care patients had significantly fewer emergency department visits, hospital days, skilled nursing facility days, and physician visits. There was a 45% decrease in costs compared with usual care patients. A randomized study showed increased satisfaction when palliative care was added to usual care. There were fewer emergency department visits and lower costs (mean cost for patients enrolled in the palliative care group was $12,670, compared with $20,222 for usual care).[36] The palliative care approach has been adopted by many other Kaiser Permanente groups as part of routine care for patients with advanced illness. Nationally, palliative care has demonstrated the ability to save hospitals significant amounts of money while delivering excellent appropriate care. Based on this experience, if New York Medicaid had palliative care services at all the New York hospitals, it would save more than $84 million a year.[37]

Teaching staff about choices for ICU use can improve economic outcomes. In one setting, an ethicist in the surgical ICU addressed the issues of patient choice about dying and the ethics of futile care. The project involved giving the residents increased knowledge and skills in addressing and integrating practical ethical issues into their surgical resident practice.[38] This was associated with a decrease in length of stay from 28 to 16 days and a decrease in surgical intensive care days from 2,028 to 1,003, far greater than observed in other parts of the hospital. Cost savings were estimated at $1.8 million. In a similar project, Dowdy and colleagues performed proactive ethics consultations for all mechanically ventilated patients beyond four days and showed improved length of stay (less use of the ICU, either by discontinuing futile care or transferring the patient to lesser intensity units) and a decrease in costs.[39] In general, consultations with an expert team work better than training the existing staff in palliative care.

Clinical practice guidelines for cancer patients now recommend concurrent palliative care as part of comprehensive cancer care. In 2012, the American Society of Clinical Oncology issued a provisional clinical opinion that recommended all patients with metastatic non–small cell lung cancer be offered palliative care, at the time of diagnosis, along with standard cancer therapy. The opinion further stated that palliative care should be considered early in the course of cancer for any patient with other metastatic cancers, as well as for those with a high burden of cancer-related symptoms.[39]

Several studies have demonstrated that utilizing palliative care improves quality while reducing cost. Other data suggest that hospice care can be cost saving. Hospice enrollment during the longer period of 53 to 105 days before death, and during the most common period of within 30 days before death, lowers Medicare expenditures, rates of hospital and ICU use, 30-day hospital readmissions, and in-hospital deaths.[40,41] In a retrospective study of 12,000 patients at 40 centers, Aiken[42] found that hospice patients were more likely to receive home nursing care and to spend less time in the hospital than conventional care patients. Of the three models of care evaluated, conventional care was the least expensive, when overall disease-management costs were calculated, but hospital-based hospice ($2,270) and home care hospice ($2,657) were less expensive than conventional care ($6,100) in the last month of life.

Advance Directives

Current studies show only 0% to 10% healthcare cost savings when individuals have advance directives. Treatment-limiting advance directives were associated with lower probabilities of in-hospital death in high- and medium-spending regions of our country, but not in low-spending regions. Cost is believed to be driven by physician practice style, rather than by differences in patients' preferences for aggressiveness of treatment at the end of life. Of note, only one in five Americans has completed a living will, and in many cases, by the time the family decides that the living will applies, the end is indeed close (a few days), and most funds have been spent. We have missed the opportunity to put hospice in place at home, so the person dies in the hospital—not what the person wanted, and at great expense. Advance directives, such as do-not-resuscitate (DNR) orders, have been advocated to allow patients to make autonomous choices about their care at the end of life and possibly to reduce costs by preventing futile care. Often, healthcare providers do not discuss goals of care with patients who have a life-limiting disease. Determining what "futile medical care" is and when to withhold it raises an important point: Even if the patient and family, at the end of life, refuse life-sustaining intervention, the patient may not require less care, but rather care of a different kind, which may be just as expensive. In fact, one retrospective from Germany purports that patients who had a palliative care consultation, compared with those who did not, were more likely to get opiates but also to die in the hospital, and cost more.[42] Despite a belief that the use of advance directives and hospice care, along with reducing futile medical care, can save our health system money, only 3.3% ($69 billion) of all health spending could actually be saved by using such practices.[43] But importantly, improvements in end of life care would not cost extra.

Nursing Issues

As healthcare reform evolves, nurses have the ability to affect clinical intervention while promoting appropriate use of resources. Nurses play a large role in the decisions patients, families, and other healthcare providers make, and those decisions drive the cost of care. Role utilization and its potential influence will vary within each setting. For example, a complete interdisciplinary palliative care team may be necessary to meet the needs of the population in a large university-based hospital, yet a specially trained nurse with interdisciplinary support may be adequate in a small community hospital. Such coupling of services should be examined from the standpoint of quality of care and cost effectiveness.[44] Advanced practice nurses may play a significant role in identifying and coordinating the needs of patients and families requiring palliation. Advanced practice nurses are perfectly positioned to fill such a critical need for this population in the hospital, hospice, and nursing home.

A factor not fully examined is the out-of-pocket cost that the patient's significant others bear in caring for them. These include lost work hours, expended resources, and simple care hours, not reimbursed through insurance or government assistance. Also to be determined is the increased healthcare costs of those caregivers, who frequently neglect their own health while caring for others.

Nursing as a profession needs to continue to advocate for this population while supporting effective quality care and fair utilization of resources. The use of advanced technology, especially expensive diagnostic tests, may be accepted as routine in an acute care hospital, regardless of cost and goals of care. Nurses must be knowledgeable about healthcare outcomes, in particular, those issues related to palliative care: the patient and family unit of care, quality of life, and decision-making about end of life care. Unfortunately, many nurses are largely unaware of and/or uninformed about these issues. Those that are aware may not have a voice within their institutions. Greater knowledge may empower nurses to take a more prominent, collaborative place at the table when such issues are being discussed and decisions are being made.

Conclusion

Economic outcomes are increasingly important for all types of healthcare, including palliative care. There are substantial opportunities for improvement using disease-management strategies and care pathways. Directed, ethically motivated interventions about futile medical care appear to produce significant cost savings. The use of advance directives or hospice care may be good medical care but has not been shown to produce major economic benefit. Most recently, integrated palliative care teams have been shown to reduce hospital and end of life care costs for seriously ill patients.

The cost of healthcare is rising because of the increasing age of the population, more cancer cases and chronic diseases, increased demand for treatment, and new and expensive technologies. Our limited resources must be rationed wisely so that we can provide both curative and palliative care. The ethical implications of using economic and management outcomes, rather than traditional health outcomes, include shifting emphasis from helping at all cost to helping at a cost society can afford, as well as determining how much society is willing to pay. The value of care to the dying versus those with curable illnesses and the tolerance of suboptimal care are ethical and societal issues.

From the perspective of economics and health service research, the outcomes of palliative care do not differ from those of other cancer treatment or from those of treatment of other chronic illnesses. For treatment to be justified, there must be some demonstrable improvement in disease-free or overall survival, toxicity, quality of life, or cost-effectiveness. Palliative care may improve survival, but it does not have a measurable cost-effectiveness ratio because it does not usually gain years of life.

Nurses clearly have the ability to affect the quality and cost of care for patients with life-limiting illness and should be at the forefront of these issues. Economic issues are critical, and nursing is in a position to make an impact. The final caveat will, however, always be to do the right thing.

References

1. Centers for Medicare and Medicaid Services, Office of the Actuary, National Health Statistics group, *National Health Care Expenditures Data*. January 2012. http://www.cms.gov/Research-Statistics-Data-and-Systems/Statistics-Trends-and-Reports/NationalHealthExpendData/index.html?redirect=/nationalhealthexpenddata/. Accessed October 27, 2014.

2. Robert Wood Johnson Foundation. *High and Rising Health Care Costs: Demystifying U.S. Health Care Spending.* October 2008. http://www.rwjf.org/content/dam/farm/reports/reports/2008/rwjf32703. Accessed October 27, 2014.

3. Centers for Medicare and Medicaid Services. *Projections of National Health Expenditures, Methodology and Model Specifications.* Available at: https://www.cms.gov/Research-Statistics-Data-and-Systems/Statistics-Trends-and-Reports/NationalHealthExpendData/downloads/projections-methodology.pdf. Accessed October 27, 2014.

4. Kaiser Family Foundation and Health Research and Educational Trust. *Employer Health Benefits 2012 Annual Survey.* September 2012. http://kff.org/private-insurance/report/employer-health-benefits-2012-annual-survey/. Accessed October 27, 2014.

5. Kaiser Family Foundation. *Medicare Chartbook, 2010.* http://kff.org/medicare/report/medicare-chartbook-2010. Accessed October 8, 2014.

6. Meier DE, Isaacs SL, Hughes R, eds. *Palliative Care: Transforming the Care of Serious Illness*. Robert Wood Johnson Foundation Health Policy Series. San Francisco: Jossey-Bass; 2010.

7. Martin AB, Lassman D, Washington B, Catlin A; National Health Expenditure Accounts Team. Growth in US health spending remained slow in 2010; health share of gross domestic product was unchanged from 2009. *Health Affairs*. 2012;31(1):208–219.

8. Kelly A, McGarry K, Fahle S, eds. Out-of-pocket spending in the last five years of life. *J Gen Intern Med*. 2013;28(2):304–309.

9. Woolhandler S, Himmelstein D, Adams G, Almberg M. Despite slight drop in uninsured, last year's figure points to 48,000 preventable deaths. Physicians for a National Health Program. September 12, 2012.

10. Children's Defense Fund. www.childrensdefense.org. Accessed October 8, 2014.

11. Riley GF, Lubitz JD. Long-term trends in medicare payments in the last year of life. *Health Services Res*. 2010;45:565–576.

12. Teno JM, Gozalo PL, Bynum JPW, et al. Change in end of life care for medicare beneficiaries: site of death, place of care, and healthcare transitions in 2000, 2005, and 2009. *JAMA*. 2013;309:470.

13. Kelley AS, McGarry K, Fahle S, Marshall SM. Out-of-pocket spending in the last five years of life. *J Gen Intern Med*. 2013;28:304–309.

14. SUPPORT Principal Investigators. A controlled trial to improve care for seriously ill hospitalized patients. The Study to Understand Prognoses and Preferences for Outcomes and Risks of Treatments (SUPPORT). *JAMA*. 1995;274:1591–1598.

15. Cohen MZ, Easley MK, Ellis C, et al. for the JCAHO. Cancer pain management and the JCAHO's Pain Standards: an institutional challenge. *J Pain Symptom Manage*. 2003;25:519–527.

16. Deandrea S, Montanari M, Moja L, Apolone G. Prevalence of undertreatment in cancer pain: a review of published literature *Ann Oncol*. 2008;19(12):1985–1991.

17. Fisch MJ, Lee JW, Weiss M, et al. Prospective, observational study of pain and analgesic prescribing in medical oncology outpatients with breast, colorectal, lung, or prostate cancer. *J Clin Oncol*. 2012;30(16):1980–1988.

18. Frist W. How do you want to die? 2012. http://theweek.com//bullpen/column/233111/how-do-you-want-to-die. Accessed October 8, 2014.

19. Centers for Disease Control and Prevention. Infant health. 2010. http://www.cdc.gov/nchs/fastats/infant-health.htm. Accessed October 8, 2014.

20. Parikh RB, Kirch R, Smith TJ, Temel J. Early specialty palliative care: translating data in oncology into practice and policy. *N Engl J Med*. 2013;369(24):2347–2351

21. Harrington SE, Smith TJ. The role of chemotherapy at the end of life: "when is enough, enough?" *JAMA*. 2008;299(22):2667–2678.

22. Berger JT, Rosner F. The ethics of practice guidelines. *Arch Intern Med*. 1996;156:2051–2056.

23. Callahan D. Controlling the costs of healthcare for the elderly: fair means and foul. *N Engl J Med*. 1996;335:744–746.

24. Randall F. *Palliative Care Ethics: A Good Companion*. New York, NY: Oxford University Press; 1996.

25. Daniels N. *Just Health Care*. New York, NY: Cambridge University Press; 1985.

26. Sidgwick H. *The Methods of Ethics*. London: McMillan; 1907.

27. Center for the Advancement of Palliative Care. CAPC state by state report card [serial online]. 2011. http://www.capc.org/reportcard/. Accessed October 27, 2014.

28. Trowman R, Chung H, Longson C, et al. The National Institute for Health and Clinical Excellence and its role in assessing the value of new cancer treatments in England and Wales. *Clin Cancer Res*. 2011;17(15):4930–4935.

29. Matsuyama R, Reddy S, Smith TJ. Why do patients choose chemotherapy near the end of life? A review of the perspective of those facing death from cancer. *J Clin Oncol*. 2006;24(21):3490–3496.

30. Slevin ML, Stubbs L, Plant HJ, et al. Attitudes to chemotherapy: comparing views of patients with cancer with those of doctors, nurses, and general public. *BMJ*. 1990;300:1458–1460.

31. http://www.oecd.org. Accessed October 27, 2014.

32. Smith TJ, Hillner BE, Desch CE. Efficacy and cost-effectiveness of cancer treatment: rational allocation of resources based on decision analysis. *J Natl Cancer Inst*. 1993;85:1460–1474.

33. Laupacis A, Feeny D, Detsky AS, Tugwell PX. How attractive does a new technology have to be to warrant adoption and utilization? Tentative guidelines for using clinical and economic evaluation. *Can Med Assoc J*. 1992;146:473–481.

34. Smith TJ. Which hat do I wear? *JAMA*. 1993;270:1657–1659.

35. Higginson IJ, Costantini M, Silber E, et al. Evaluation of a new model of short-term palliative care for people severely affected with multiple sclerosis: a randomised fast-track trial to test timing of referral and how long the effect is maintained. *Postgrad Med J*. 2011;87:769–775.

36. Swetz KM, Smith TJ. Palliative chemotherapy: when is it worth it and when is it not? *Cancer J*. 2010;16(5):467–472.

37. Brumley R, Enguidanos S, Jamison P, et al. Increased satisfaction with care and lower costs: results of a randomized trial of in-home palliative care. *J Am Geriatr Soc*. 2007;55(7):993–1000.

38. Morrison RS, Dietrich J, Ladwig S, et al. Palliative care consultation teams cut hospital costs for medicaid beneficiaries. *Health Affairs*. 2011;30: 454–463.

39. Dowdy MD, Robertson C, Bander JA. A study of proactive ethics consultation for critically and terminally ill patients with extended lengths of stay. Crit Care Med 1998;26:252–259.

40. Smith TJ, Temin S, Alesi E, et al. American Society of Clinical Oncology provisional clinical opinion: the integration of palliative care into standard oncology care. *J Clin Oncol*. 2012;30(8):880–887.

41. Kelley AS, Partha D, Qingling D, et al. The CARE SPAN hospice enrollment saves money for Medicare and improves care quality across a number of different lengths-of-stay. *Health Affairs*. 2013;32(3):552–561.

42. Aiken LS, Butner J, Lockhart CA, et al. Outcome evaluation of a randomized trial of the PhoenixCare intervention: program of case management and coordinated care for the seriously chronically ill. *J Palliat Med.* 2006;9(1):111–126.

43. Gaertner J, Drabik A, Marschall U, et al. Inpatient palliative care: a nationwide analysis. *Health Policy.* 2013;109(3):311–318.

44. Emanuel EJ. Cost savings at the end of life: what do the data show? *JAMA.* 1996;275(24):1907–1914.

45. Coyne PJ. The case of Mrs. A. *J Palliat Med.* 2012;15(12):1397–1398.

Appendix I

Sample CQI Study Proposal to Improve End of Life Care Using FOCUS-PCAD[i]

*F*ind *a process to improve.*

Set the boundaries by defining the beginning and end points of the process.

Opportunity statement
An opportunity exists to improve <u>EOL care for the imminently dying inpatient,</u>
(Name the process.)
beginning with <u>a physicians' order for the Palliative Care for Advanced Disease care path</u>
ending with <u>death or discharge to homecare, hospice, or residential facility.</u>
(Set boundaries.)
This effort should improve <u>patient comfort and family satisfaction with EOL care</u>
(Name outcome measure)
for <u>hospitalized oncology, geriatric, hospice, and intensive care unit patients.</u>
(Name the customers.)

The process is important to work on now because <u>good EOL care is an institutional priority, no benchmarks are currently available in the US, and no standard approach is used at BIMC* to assess and treat patients who are imminently dying.</u>
(State significance.)

*O*rganize *to improve the process.*

Form a multidisciplinary CQI team; establish roles, rules, and meeting times.

Multidisciplinary Team (22 members)
Department of Pain Medicine and Palliative Care
MDs, nurses, social workers, psychologist, chaplain
Hospital departments
Ethics
Pediatrics
Nutrition
Quality improvement
Pharmacy
Outcomes measurement (research grants and contracts)
Pilot units (Oncology, Geriatrics, Intensive Care, Hospice)
Nurse managers, case managers, clinical nurse specialists

———
* BIMC: Beth Israel Medical Center

131

[i] Reprinted with permission from Bookbinder MB, Blank AE, Arney E, et al. Improving End of Life-Care: Development and Pilot Test of Clinical Pathway. J Pain Symptom Manage, (2005) Jun; 29(6): 529–43.

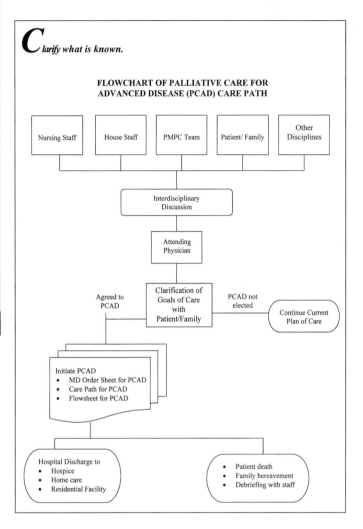

*C*larify what is known.

FLOWCHART OF PALLIATIVE CARE FOR
ADVANCED DISEASE (PCAD) CARE PATH

Nursing Staff | House Staff | PMPC Team | Patient/ Family | Other Disciplines

Interdisciplinary Discussion

Attending Physician

Clarification of Goals of Care with Patient/Family

Agreed to PCAD

PCAD not elected

Continue Current Plan of Care

Initiate PCAD
- MD Order Sheet for PCAD
- Care Path for PCAD
- Flowsheet for PCAD

Hospital Discharge to
- Hospice
- Home care
- Residential Facility

- Patient death
- Family bereavement
- Debriefing with staff

Understand the variation

Brainstorm with those at the grass roots level about why the process varies. Categorize sources of variation by people, materials, methods, and equipment. Display data using a cause-and-effect diagram.

Brainstorming Session with CQI Team on End-of-life (EOL) Care Question:
What barriers could be encountered in implementing an EOL Pathway at BIMC?

EOL awareness/ discomfort/readiness:

What is "end-of-life care?" When is treatment palliative vs. life ending? How do we choose?
Patient, family, readiness/awareness of dying
Physician, family, patient willingness to acknowledge that death is imminent
Issues of truth-telling: family may not know status of patient prior to the pathway
Physician discomfort with stopping treatment
Medical uncertainty about when to stop treatment

Team communication:

Physician and nurse discomfort in discussing change in treatment strategy
Is it the physician's decision alone? The heath care team as a whole needs to be acknowledged in decision.
Definition of terms. Need to define who the team is. May need a new model.
Nurses' comfort—may be put in the middle of team/family attending and decisions.

Unit resistance:

Resistance of unit teams. May see this project as "another thing to do."
Large-scale resistance. Some may not see that there is something to "fix."
Organizational pressure to discharge quickly.

Knowledge deficit:

Assumptions about pastoral care (patient, family, staff) and what the experience will be.
Knowledge deficit about medical and nursing interventions
How to implement the care path and encourage people to speak upfront rather than later
Large cultural diversity at BIMC
Education needed about biomedical analysis and ethical problems
Physician/patient and physician/family communication skills

Cause and Effect (Ishikawa) Diagram (Barriers to implementing PCAD)—Themes above

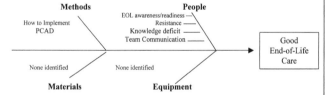

Select the process improvement.

Describe the new intervention in detail. Palliative Care for Advanced Disease (PCAD) Care Path: Care Path, Flow Sheet, and Physicians' Order Sheet **(see following pages)**

BETH ISRAEL HEALTH CARE SYSTEM	☐ PETRIE DIVISION	☐ NORTH DIVISION	☐ KINGS HWY DIVISION
Care Path: *PALLIATIVE CARE for ADVANCED DISEASE*	PRE-ADMISSION CONSIDERATION/ ADMISSION CRITERIA ☐ Disease at Advanced Stage – limited life expectancy ____ ☐ HCP: Agent ____ ☐ DNR ☐ Primary Caregiver ____ ☐ Next of Kin ____	DISCHARGE OUTCOMES ☐ Discharge to Community: – Hospice _ Home Care – Alternative Care Facility _Home or ☐ Patient expired/Bereavement resources provided to family	STAMP ADDRESSOGRAPH NAME OF SERVICE/ATTENDING/ HOUSE MD
PLAN:	START DATE:		ONGOING DAYS:
TREATMENTS/ INTERVENTIONS/ ASSESSMENTS	1) CLARIFY GOALS OF PALLIATIVE CARE FOR ADVANCED DISEASE (PCAD) WITH PATIENT AND/OR FAMILY 2) FACILITATE DISCUSSION & DOCUMENTATION OF ADVANCE DIRECTIVES: Identify designated individuals & roles in decision-making: 1) Health Care Agent 3) Primary Caregiver 2) Durable Power of Attorney 4) Next-of-kin Identify patient/family preferences regarding: • Health Care Proxy • Resuscitation Status/DNR • Living Will 3) INITIATE PHYSICIAN ORDER SHEET/REVIEW DAILY 4) COMFORT ASSESSMENT to include • Pain and symptom management needs • Psychosocial coping, anticipatory grieving, and social/cultural needs • Spiritual issues and distress 5) VS – None unless useful in promoting pt/family comfort 6) ASSESS FOR AND PROVIDE ENVIRONMENT CONDUCIVE TO MEET PATIENT & FAMILY NEEDS		REPEAT CARE PATH DAILY DOCUMENT IN: DAILY PATIENT CARE FLOW SHEET PROGRESS NOTES
PAIN MANAGEMENT	1) ASSESS PAIN Q 4 HR and evaluate within 1 hr post intervention. Complete pain assessment scale. Anticipate pain needs.		
TESTS/PROCEDURES	1) USUALLY UNNECESSARY for patient/family comfort (All lab work and diagnostic work is discouraged)		
MEDICATIONS	1) Medication regimen focus is the RELIEF OF DISTRESSING SYMPTOMS.		
FLUIDS/NUTRITION	1) DIET: Selective diet with no restrictions • Nutrition to be guided by patient's choice of time, place, quantities and type of food desired. Family may provide food. • Educate family in nutritional needs of dying patient 2) IVs for symptom management only 3) TRANSFUSIONS for symptom relief only 4) INTAKE AND OUTPUT – consider goals of care relative to patient comfort 5) WEIGHTS – consider risks/benefits relative to patient comfort		

©Continuum Health Partners, Inc., Department of Pain Medicine & Palliative Care 1999

ACTIVITY	1) ACTIVITY DETERMINED BY PATIENT'S PREFERENCES AND ABILITY. Patient determines participation in ADLs, i.e., turning and positioning, bathing, transfers	REPEAT CARE PATH DAILY DOCUMENT IN: DAILY PATIENT CARE FLOW SHEET PROGRESS NOTES
CONSULTS	1) INITIATE referrals to institutional specialists to optimize comfort and enhance quality of life (QOL) only.	

PSYCHOSOCIAL NEEDS	1) PSYCHOSOCIAL COMFORT ASSESSMENT of:
	  • Patient
	  • Primary caregiver
	  • Grieving process of patient & family
	
	2) PSYCHOSOCIAL SUPPORT: Referral to Social Work
	  • Offer emotional support
	  • Support verbalization and anticipatory grieving
	  • Encourage family caring activities as appropriate/individualized to family situation and culture
	  • Facilitate verbal and tactile communication
	  • Assist family with nutrition, transportation, child care, financial, funeral issues
	  • Assess bereavement needs	

SPIRITUAL NEEDS	1) SPIRITUAL COMFORT ASSESSMENT
	  • Spiritual supports
	  • Spiritual needs and/or distress
	
	2) SPIRITUAL SUPPORT: Referral to Chaplain
	  • Provide opportunity for expression of beliefs, fears, and hopes
	  • Provide access to religious resources
	  • Facilitate religious practices	

PATIENT/FAMILY EDUCATION	1) ASSESS NEEDS AND PROVIDE EDUCATION REGARDING:
	  • Goals of Palliative Care for Advanced Disease
	  • Physical and psychosocial needs during the dying process
	  • Coping techniques/Relaxation techniques
	  • Bereavement process and resources	

DISCHARGE PLANNING	1) FOR DISCHARGE TO COMMUNITY: Referral to Pain Medicine & Palliative Care/ Hospice/Home Care/Social Work as needed.
	
	2) AT TIME OF DEATH:
	  • Post Mortem care observing cultural and religious practices and preferences
	  • Provide for care of patient's possessions as per family wishes
	  • Bereavement support for family and staff	

©Continuum Health Partners, Inc., Department of Pain Medicine & Palliative Care 1999

This document is to be used as a guideline only. Each case should be evaluated and treated individually based upon clinical findings.

Appendix II

Carepath: Palliative Care for Advanced Disease[i]

This document is to be used as a guideline only. Each case should be evaluated and treated individually based upon clinical findings.

Beth Israel Health Care System
Carepath: Palliative Care for Advanced Disease
DAILY PATIENT CARE FLOW SHEET

ADDRESSOGRAPH

DATE:

☐ DNR ☐ NO DNR ☐ HCP ☐ NO HCP HCP AGENT: CAREGIVER:

COMFORT ASSESSMENT: Comfort Level Patient states or appears to be
1. Always comfortable 2. Usually comfortable 3. Sometimes comfortable 4. Seldom comfortable 5. Never comfortable

TIME (per MD order)									
PATIENT Comfort Level (Indicate number)									
VITAL SIGNS ONLY AS ORDERED — T									
P									
R									
BP									

PAIN/RELIEF SCALE KEY
NONE — WORST
0 1 2 3 4 5 6 7 8 9 10
COMPLETE RELIEF — NO RELIEF

SEDATION SCALE
0 Alert
1 Awake but drowsy
2 Drowsy/Easily awakened
3 Sleeping/Easily awakened
4 Sleeping/Difficult to awaken
5 Unarousable

PAIN	TIME									
	LOCATION									
	PAIN RATING									
	RELIEF/SEDATION									

* See Progress Note   A = Assessment   I = Intervention   Check mark = present or done   * Needs MD Order

		Time						Time						Time		
EYES	A	Moist/Clear				**BREATHING**	A	Rate: Normal				**NUTRITION**	A	Full meal		
		Inflamed						Rapid						> 50%		
		Dry/Crusted						Slow						< 50%		
								Rhythm: Reg						Refused		
								Irregular						Nausea/vomiting		
	I	Routine Care						Depth: Normal						NPO		
		Artificial Tears						Shallow						Dysphagia		
		Oint/Lubricant						Labored								
								Secretions: None					I	Diet as tolerated		
LIPS	A	Smooth/moist						Mild						NG/G tube		
		Dry/Cracked						Copious						Enteral feeding		
		Ulcerated						Breath sounds:						Feeding set changed		
								Clear						Residual vol-cc's		
	I	Routine Care						Diminished						Placement check		
		Topical Lubricant						Absent						Meds as ordered		
								Crackles								
								Wheeze					IV	IV site		
MOUTH	A	Moist						Dyspnea					A	No S&S infil/phleb		
		Dry					I	None						Dry & intact		
		Coated						Reposition					I	IV Dsg change		
		Stomatitis						O2 via ___ @ ___ lpm						IV Tubing change		
								Suctioning q						See progress note		
								Trach Care						Cap Change		
	I	Routine Care						Elevate HOB						Huber needle change		
		*Artificial Saliva						Fan								
		Magic Wash						Meds as ordered								
		Meds as ordered														

[i] Reprinted with permission from Bookbinder MB, Blank AE, Arney E, et al. Improving End of Life-Care: Development and Pilot Test of Clinical Pathway. J Pain Symptom Manage, (2005) Jun; 29(6): 529–43.

		Time							Time							Time		
M	**A**	Bedbound				**S**	**A**	Normal				**F**	**A**	Engaged w pt		
O		OOB Chair				**L**		Interrupted Cycle				**A**		Coping w loss		
B		Amb w Assist				**E**		Insomnia				**M**		Distressed		
I		OOB ad lib				**E**						**I**				
L		BR Privileges				**P**	**I**	Modify Environment				**L**				
I	**I**	T&P per pt comfort						Relaxation				**Y**	**I**	Goals of care reviewed		
T		ROM q						Meds as order						Encourage verbal		
Y		Assistive Device												& non-verbal		
		__ Ted Stocking(s)				**P**	**A**	Awake/alert						communication w pt		
		Side Rails Up				**S**		Responds to voice						Family Meeting		
E	**A**	Voiding qs				**Y**		Resp to tactile stim						Bereavement		
L		Anuria				**C**		Unresponsive						support		
I		Incontinent Urine				**H**		Oriented								
M		Bowel Movement				**O**		Confused								
I		Incontinent Feces				**S**		Hallucinating								
N		Diarrhea				**O**		Calm								
A		Constipation				**C**		Anxiety				**M**		AM Care		
T						**I**		Agitated				**I**		PM Care		
I	**I**	__ Foley Catheter				**A**		Depression				**S**		PresUlcer Prev Plan		
O		Texas Catheter				**L**		Spiritual distress				**C**		Fall Prev Plan		
N		Inc't Pads										**E**		Precautions:		
		__ Enema					**I**	Emotional support				**L**		Isolation:		
		Meds as ordered						Verbal/tactile				**L**		Siderails Up		
								stimulation				**A**		ID Bracelet		
								Social Worker visit				**N**		Allergy Bracelet		
S	**A**	Normal/Intact						Chaplain visit				**E**		DNR Bracelet		
K		Feverish										**O**		Post Mortem care		
I		Diaphoretic										**U**				
N		Pressure Ulcer Stg__										**S**				
		Ostomy site D/I						Comments/Progress Notes								
		Edema														
		Pruritis														
		Cool/Mottled														
W	**I**	Site														
O		Dressing____														
U		Dry & Intact														
N		Drain____														
D		Drainage														
		Odor														
C		Ostomy site care														
A		Tube site care														
R																
E																

PATIENT/FAMILY EDUCATION: See IPFER

PCAD Care Path: Initiated Reviewed/Continue With Plan Of Care ☐ Revised (See Progress Note)

OTHER NURSING DOCUMENTATION:
☐ I & O SHEET ☐ RESTRAINT FLOW SHEET ☐ NEURO-ASSESSMENT ☐ OTHER_____

SIGNATURE/TITLE	DATE	SHIFT	INITIALS	SIGNATURE/TITLE	DATE	SHIFT	INITIALS
1.				6.			
2.				7.			
3.				8.			
4.				9.			
5.				10.			

Beth Israel Health Care System
DOCTOR'S ORDER SHEET
PALLIATIVE CARE FOR ADVANCED DISEASE

ADMISSION HT_____   ADMISSION WEIGHT_____

ADDRESSOGRAPH AREA

ORDERS OTHER THAN MEDICATION/INFUSION	MEDICATION/INFUSION (Specify route & directions)
1 Primary Diagnosis:	1. Assess patient for the following symptoms:
2 Activate PCAD Care Path	Anxiety & Insomnia Hiccups
3 Anticipated time on PCAD Care Path:	Confusion/Agitation Nausea/Vomiting
___ hours ___days ___weeks ___unknown	Constipation Pain
	Depressed Mood Pruritis
4 Allergies:	Diarrhea Stomatitis
5 Diet: □ No restrictions (food may be provided by caregiver)	Dyspnea Terminal Secretions
□ NPO □ Other:	Fever (Noisy Respirations)
	See reverse side for suggestions for pain management
6 Activity: □ OOB as tolerated □ OOB with assistance	*and symptom control*
7 Vital Signs: □ Discontinue	2. DISCONTINUE ALL PREVIOUS MED ORDERS
□ Daily □ q shift □ q ___hours	3. ORDERS:
8 Comfort Assessment: □q __ hr □q 2 hr □q 4 hr □q shift	
9 Weight: □ None □ q ____ day(s)	
10 I & O: □ None q _____	
11 Visiting: □ Open visiting, nurse-restrictions apply	
□ Per routine policy	
□ Other:	
12 DNR: □ Yes □ No	
13 PCAD Care Path will include (specify if otherwise):	
Psychosocial Care – Social Work Referral	
Spiritual Care – Chaplaincy Referral	
14 Consults:	
□ Pain Medicine & Palliative Care Consult	
□ Ethics Consult	
□ Hospice Consult	
□ Other:	
15 Labs: □ Discontinue all previous standing orders	
□ Continue previous lab orders	
□ Other labs:	
16 Oxygen Therapy: _____L/min via_____	
17 Other orders:	

CLERK	DATE	TIME	NURSE'S SIGNATURE	PRESCRIBER'S SIGNATURE	ID#	DATE	TIME

©Continuum Health Partners, Inc., Department of Pain Medicine & Palliative Care 1999

The following are medications for consideration in treating pain and symptoms of patients on PCAD:

PAIN MANAGEMENT
For Opioid-Naïve Patient:
Morphine Sulfate 15 mg po or 5 mg SQ/IV.
Repeat q 1 hr until pain relief is adequate. Begin Morphine Sulfate 30 mg po or 10 mg SQ/IV q 4 hr ATC or begin IV Morphine Sulfate basal infusion at 2 mg per hour and 2 mg SQ/IV q 1 hr prn.

For Opioid-Treated Patient:
If pain uncontrolled, increase fixed schedule dose by 50%.

Many non-opioid analgesics are available and should be considered after opioid therapy has been optimized. If pain remains uncontrolled, consider consult to Department of Pain Medicine and Palliative Care (Beeper #6702).

ANXIETY & INSOMNIA
Lorazepam 0.5mg po/SQ/IV BID-TID q HS for anxiety.
Temazepam 15 – 30 mg po q HS for anxiety/ insomnia.
Clonazepam 0.5 – 2 mg po BID-TID for anxiety/myoclonus.

CONFUSION/AGITATION
Haloperidol 0.5 mg po/SQ/IV. Repeat q 30 minutes until symptom intensity declines.
Haloperidol 0.5 – 5 mg po/SQ/IV q 4 hr prn.

CONSTIPATION
Lactulose 30 ml po q 2 hr prn until constipation relieved.
When symptom improves, begin Lactulose 30 ml po q 12 hr.
Warm Fleets Enema TIW prn

To prevent constipation:
Senokot 1 – 2 tabs po BID and
Colace 1 – 2 tabs po BID.

SYMPTOMS OF DEPRESSION
If anticipated survival is in weeks:
Begin SSRI, e.g., Paroxetine 20 mg po daily, and titrate to effect.

If anticipated survival is in days:
Methylphenidate 2.5 mg po q morning and at noon and escalate daily to 5 – 10 mg po q morning and at noon or Pemoline 18.75 mg po q morning and at noon and escalate daily to 37.5 mg po q morning and at noon.
Higher doses may be needed.

Consider Liaison Psychiatry consultation

DIARRHEA
Loperamide 4 mg po q 4 hr prn

DYSPNEA
For Opioid-Naïve Patient:
Morphine Sulfate 5 – 15 mg po or 2 – 5 mg SQ/IV. Repeat q 1 hr, if needed. When symptom is improved, begin Morphine Sulfate 30 mg po or 10 mg SQ/IV q 4 hr ATC; or begin Morphine Sulfate basal infusion at 2 mg per hour and 2 mg SQ/IV q 1 hr prn.

For Opioid-Treated Patient:
If dyspnea uncontrolled, increase fixed schedule dose by 50%.
If breathlessness continues, add Lorazepam 0.5mg po or SQ/IV prn. Repeat q 60 minutes if needed until symptom intensity declines, then begin 1 mg po/SQ/IV q 3 hr.

Additional therapies may include:
Dexamethasone 16 mg po/IV, followed by 4 mg po/IV q 6 hr
Albuterol 2.5 mg via nebulization q 4 hr prn if wheezing present

FEVER
Acetaminophen 650 mg po/PR q 4 hr prn, and/or
Dexamethasone 1.0 mg po/SQ/IV q 12 hr prn

HICCUPS
Chlorpromazine 10 – 25 mg po/IM TID prn
Haloperidol 0.5 – 2 mg po/SQ/IV TID – QID

INTRACTABLE SYMPTOMS, MANAGEMENT OF
Consider referral to Department of Pain Medicine & Palliative Care (Beeper # 6702).

IV HYDRATION
Consider decreasing IV rate to 0.5 – 1 liter/24 hr

NAUSEA/VOMITING
Metoclopramide 10 mg po/IV q 4 hr prn, or
Prochlorperazine 10 mg po/IV q 4 hr or 25 mg PR q 8 hr prn with or without Dexamethasone 4 mg po/IVPB q 6 hr

PRURITIS
Diphenhydramine 25 – 50 mg po/IV q 12 hr
Hydrocortisone 1 % cream to affected areas q 6 hr
Dexamethasone 1.0 mg po daily alone or in combination with above

STOMATITIS
Viscous lidocaine 2 % to painful areas prn
Clotrimazole 10 mg troche 5 times daily
Nystatin S & S q 6 hr prn
Magic Mouthwash prn

TERMINAL SECRETIONS (NOISY RESPIRATIONS)
Scopolamine patches 1.5 – 3 mg 72 hr, or
Scopolamine 0.4 mg SQ q 4 – 6 hr

PLAN—DO—CHECK—ACT (the Shewhart cycle)

$\boldsymbol{P}_{lan}$

Create a timeline of resources, activities, training, and target dates. Develop a data collection plan, the tools for measuring outcomes, and thresholds for determining when targets have been met.

Timeline for One-Year Pilot CQI EOL Project

Phase 0 – Planning

Jan – June	Formalize CQI Team for the development of a clinical pathway.
	Clarify knowledge of processes: review literature and existing data sources, conduct brainstorming, flowcharting with pilot units.
	Evaluate and synthesize literature, tools, other data gathered.
	Identify content for Care Path.
	Develop and pilot audit tool for chart reviews.
	Create database, codebook, and scoring guidelines for data entry.
	Identify patient outcome assessment tools.
	Identify family outcome assessment tools.
	Identify staff assessment tools.
	Refine study tools/procedures.
	Develop staff education.
	Develop caregiver educational materials.
June 21	Medical Records review
Aug 2	Tools Committee review
July 3	Committee on Scientific OSA Application and Approval

Phase I – Launching the Project

August 2	Meet with hospital leadership—Introduction to Palliative Care for Advanced Disease Care Path
	• PCAD Care Path, MD Orders, and Flow sheet
	• Timeline for Education/Evaluation
August 11	Introduction of PCAD Care Path to medical staff

Phase II – Unit Implementation and Education of PCAD Care Path

	Cohort 1	Cohort 2		Cohort 3
• Meet with unit leaders of pilot units	June 21	September 15	July 21	October 11
• Pre-test	August 23–25	September 27	September 14	TBS
• Unit leadership team meeting	TBS	October 5	October 12	TBS
• Introduction of PCAD Care Path to unit staff	August 31– September 1	September 27– September 30	October 22	TBS
• In-service of unit staff	September 1 September 2 September 3	October 4– October 6	October 25– October 26	TBS TBS TBS
• Rollout of Care Path	September 6	October 11	November 1	TBS
• Brainstorming— educational needs	October 11	November 8	December 13	December 6
• Educational series	September– February	October– March	November– April	November– April
• Focus groups	October & January	November & February	December & March	December & March
• Feedback / closure / continuation	March	April	May	May
• Post-test	March	April	May	May

Phase III – Evaluation

Chart Reviews using Chart Audit Tool (CAT) (Total =330)

June–Aug	• 20 retrospective audits for 5 pilot units	(Total = 100)
Sep 1999–Mar 2002	• 20 retrospective audits for 2 control units • 10 during implementation audits for 5 pilot units • 20 post implementation audits for 5 pilot units • 20 post implementation audits for 2 control units Each patient on PCAD Care Path as admitted.	(Total = 40) (Total = 50) (Total = 100) (Total = 40)
Sep 1999–Mar 2002	Tool: Teno's After Death (interview or mailed survey)	
Dates TBD	Staff survey post-tests (4 mo post-initiation of PCAD) Tool: Palliative Care Quiz	
Sep 1999–Mar 2002	Process Audits (PAT) Ongoing throughout time patient on PCAD Care Path	
Sep 1999–Mar 2002	Brainstorming sessions and focus groups with staff to identify education 1–2 mo after each unit begins PCAD	

Phase IV – Reporting

April 15, 2002	Report to grant agency, hospital, and unit staff

Index

Page numbers followed by *f*, *t*, or *b* indicate figures, tables, or boxes, respectively.